Covid-19 Pandemic

RESPONSES AND CONSEQUENCES IN STEINER WALDORF KINDERGARTENS AND EARLY CHILDHOOD SETTINGS

Dr Neil Boland

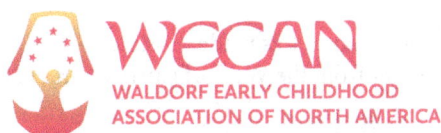

WECAN

WALDORF EARLY CHILDHOOD
ASSOCIATION OF NORTH AMERICA

Covid-19 Pandemic: Responses and consequences in Steiner Waldorf kindergartens and early childhood settings

First English Edition

ISBN: 978-1-936849-59-8

Graphic Design: Lory Widmer
Cover Image: Painting by Elisabeth Radysh

Published in the United States of America by
Waldorf Early Childhood Association of North America
285 Hungry Hollow Rd.
Spring Valley, NY 10977
www.waldorfearlychildhood.org

Visit our online store:
store.waldorfearlychildhood.org

This publication was made possible
by a grant from the Waldorf Curriculum Fund.

Contents

Index of Tables

Executive Summary

Steiner Waldorf early childhood education is represented in many countries of the world. As the international body which strives to link those who work in these different countries, IASWECE organises conferences, meetings, working groups, collaborative research projects, and training and deepening courses where people come together, united by their ideal for the development of the young child. As with so much else, any face-to-face activity was largely halted in 2020 by governmental responses to the emergence of the Covid-19 virus as countries locked down, and educational facilities had restrictions put upon them or were closed completely.

The pandemic separated us from each other, sometimes confining us to our own homes, sometimes within the areas or countries we live in when travel was restricted. Educators were separated from the children they care for, from their colleagues and from parental communities. We all know how we have been affected personally, professionally, financially, socially and health-wise by the pandemic. We know something of how those around us have been affected and gather information more widely from conversations and the media. We know that some of those in other countries have had similar or sometimes very different experiences to ourselves, but we do not always know what these are. We rarely have the opportunity to hear in detail from Waldorf colleagues around the world and learn first-hand what their experiences and challenges are. To date, there has been no overall picture available of how the worldwide Steiner early childhood movement has been affected by what is, for many of us, one of the most disruptive events in recent decades.

To respond to this, IASWECE commissioned a research project which would gather the experiences, opinions and thoughts of those who work in IASWECE member countries on the effects of the pandemic and present them in a report. It is the first time that such a large study has been undertaken of Steiner early childhood educators, and it is perhaps fitting that the topic is one which has had such worldwide impact. In this report, you will be able to hear the voices of kindergarten educators, assistants, administrators and teacher educators as they describe how they have been affected by and have responded to the challenges raised by the pandemic. Some responses will no doubt resonate with your own experiences; others may be unexpected. As a whole, they create a rich tapestry of varied experience which offers nuanced insight into the world of Steiner early childhood education as it has been practised over the last three, highly unusual years.

We hope that you will find this report interesting and that it will both broaden and deepen your understanding of the dedication and professionalism of those who work in Waldorf early childhood education and the challenges they have had to overcome.

Susan Howard and Kathy MacFarlane
For the IASWECE Council
January 2023

Introduction

The Covid-19 pandemic is one of the only truly global events which has happened in recent years and has brought an unprecedented level of disruption and uncertainty in people's daily lives, including disrupting the education of children worldwide. Due to the severe threat of the virus, governments around the world enforced strict measures, including large-scale lockdowns, travel limitations, and border closures. Governments adopted these measures to reduce close contact between individuals, including in early childhood settings and schools. Some closed educational establishments completely, others kept them open only for students with special needs or for the children of 'key workers'. How this was done varied greatly from country to country, even from state to state. Most countries closed educational facilities for at least part of the period, especially at the beginning of the pandemic; however, closures continued in many places into 2021, with restrictions continuing beyond that.

At the time of writing, the situation in most countries has returned to some kind of 'normal', though few would say that there are no lasting effects of this unprecedented and challenging period. Heightened health measures and hygiene protocols continue in some places. This report is an attempt to document the responses to and consequences of the pandemic in Steiner Waldorf early childhood settings around the world.

The project came into being through a question from Susan Howard, of the Coordinating Group of the International Association of Steiner Waldorf Early Childhood Education (IASWECE). She asked if there was any research into the experiences of Steiner early childhood educators during the Covid pandemic and the consequences for them and their centres. There is a growing body of research available into the consequences of the pandemic on young children, educators and families from a growing number of viewpoints (among others Atiles et al., 2022; Eadie et al., 2021; Lafave et al., 2022; Mitchell et al., 2020, p. 412; Souto-Manninga & Melvina, 2022; Su et al., 2022; Timmons et al., 2021), but there is none, to my knowledge, from a Steiner perspective, barring three small reports from two years ago (Boland, 2020a, 2020b; Boland & Mortlock, 2020), looking at the experiences of Australian and New Zealand educators early on in the pandemic. There are few or no studies, for instance, which look at how pedagogy was affected or which detail if changes in child development and behaviour have been noted by Steiner educators.

Following this initial contact, we began to consider how information could be gathered from IASWECE member countries and how it could be beneficial to 'take the pulse' of the movement at this stage of the pandemic. Everyone knows how the pandemic has affected them personally, professionally, socially, financially, and health-wise. Anecdotally, we know an amount from people we are in communication with, which is supplemented by accounts in the media. However, there is next to no information available on Steiner early childhood education during the pandemic period based on research rather than anecdotes, and none from a wider perspective which looks at experiences from multiple countries. It is hoped that the information in this report will allow IASWECE to plan more effectively for the future, set realistic budgets, identify and target needs, apply for external funding where needed to meet identified challenges, and have a better overall understanding of the experiences of educators widely distributed geographically but united by profession.

This was the background to the setting up of this project. So far as is known, it is the first time that information about and from Steiner Waldorf early childhood educators, including assistants, administrators and teacher educators, has been gathered from all inhabited continents, across widely different contexts. It is hoped that this study will contribute in a small way to the (limited) body of international empirical research into Steiner early childhood education. The studies which exist are on a small scale, rarely even of national scope (Attfield, 2022; de Souza, 2012; Nicol & Taplin, 2017; O'Connor, 2014; Randoll, 2015; Rawson, 2021). No international project has been attempted to take the temperature of the international early childhood body. Given that the Covid pandemic has affected every child and every teacher in the world and necessitated immediate and radical changes in pedagogy and practice, it is timely that such a study be undertaken.

This report contains a number of sections. After this introduction, the design and setting up of the study is detailed. This is followed by a description of the participants, the main findings from the responses submitted, and, lastly, a conclusion with recommendations. Copies of the surveys are included in the appendices.

Project Design

Context

Everyone has had strong experiences during the pandemic and has been affected in unique ways, substantially coloured by how each person's government responded. When one country was under a strict lockdown with kindergartens[1] closed, those in other countries were operating with few restrictions. It is beyond the scope of this small study to go into these differences in depth. The interested reader is directed towards the Oxford University Blavatnik School of Government's *Covid-19 government response tracker* (2022). This is a dynamic and helpful tool which allows evidence-based comparisons to be made of how individual governments approached the pandemic, for instance, allowing comparisons to be made of the severity of lockdowns and other restrictions imposed on early childhood settings, day by day, country by country.

The project gathered responses from the following member organisations of IASWECE:

> *Australia, Austria, Belgium, Brazil, Canada, Czech Republic, Denmark, East Africa (Kenya, Uganda, Tanzania), Estonia, Finland, France, Germany, Hungary, India, Ireland, Israel, Italy, Japan, South Korea, Lithuania, Mexico, Netherlands, New Zealand, Norway, Poland, Romania, Russia, Slovenia, South Africa, Spain, Sweden, Switzerland, Taiwan, Ukraine, United Kingdom, United States of America, and Vietnam.*

Methodology

The research project sought to gather the experiences of Steiner early childhood educators on a broad scale, across a range of countries. This data was, to a degree, time sensitive. It needed to be gathered before educators had 'forgotten' how the pandemic affected them as individuals and as educators. This was one of the main reasons why an online survey methodology was adopted.

---

1 For details of how terminology is used in this report, please see page 14.

Advantages of online questionnaires include that data can be collected quickly and easily; they do not take up a lot of the participants' time, and the quantitative data collected (using a Likert scale, in which participants chose from a set of answer options) can be analysed swiftly and made into simple-to-read graphs.

In the end, two questionnaires were designed. The first was quantitative, Likert-based (Croasmun & Ostrom, 2011) and asked questions about well-being, children's behaviours, enrolment and staffing, with a single question about vaccine mandates. This was designed to take less than five minutes to complete and was formatted so it could be answered on a mobile phone. This approach was chosen out of respect for and consideration of the time pressure many educators work under (Cumming, 2017). The second questionnaire asked four open-ended questions and sought more lengthy, detailed replies. It was expected that while (hopefully) many people would complete the first survey, a smaller number would complete the second.

The questionnaires thus involved mixed methods, being both quantitative (Likert-scale questions, able to be numerically analysed) and qualitative (open-ended questions) which were analysed thematically using a standard content analysis approach (Mayring, 2020) to identify overarching themes.

In consultation with IASWECE, the vocabulary used in the questions was plain and direct, and the questions themselves were as short as could be managed. Any specialist references would be easily understood by anyone working in the field. Loaded questions or ones leading the participant towards a certain answer were avoided (Patten, 2017). Multi-item scales were avoided because of possible display issues on some mobile phones.

Ethical considerations

As with any piece of research, it was important that strict ethical standards were maintained. To ensure these standards were met, the design of the proposed project was submitted to the Auckland University of Technology Ethics Committee (AUTEC) and which gave approval in July 2022 (#22/166).

Both questionnaires were anonymous. Data was gathered as to which country each response was being completed in (not the location, just the country) and the language it was completed in (to facilitate sorting responses). No identifying questions were asked beyond what participants' main professional role was (educator, administrator as well as educator, administrator, assistant, or teacher educator). There are so many Steiner early childhood settings, this still left participants unidentifiable. (The smallest national association of IASWECE has 10 EC settings, the largest around 600. Each employs multiple staff.)[2] Any information given by participants in Questionnaire 2 which could be identifying has been anonymised or omitted in this final report.

In order to obtain participants' consent to take part in the research, the opening screen of each questionnaire (see Appendices C and D) comprised a consent form, briefly explaining the project and making clear that continuing with the questionnaire indicated consent. Participants could leave the questionnaire at any point before the end.

In most questionnaires, care has to be taken that the selection of participants is balanced demographically, for instance by ethnicity, socioeconomic status, culture, age, and so on. Such considerations were not relevant in this study and identifying and selecting participants was straightforward. Though sizable, the number of Steiner early childhood educators is finite. The links to the questionnaires were sent to all those working in IASWECE member countries, whether as educators, assistants, administrators or teacher educators. It was expected that participants would come from a wide range of cultures and backgrounds. Inquiring into these was not a feature of the study; no identifying questions were asked about age, gender, sexuality, ethnicity, education, experience, culture, belief or similar.

In order not to compromise the integrity of the data gathering process, there was no direct contact between the researcher and participants. Instead, information was passed from the researcher to Susan Howard from the Coordinating Group of IASWECE, who in turn sent it to the national representatives on the IASWECE Council. These national representatives sent it to their member early childhood settings for distribution to all staff. Though this is a lengthy chain of communication, it was necessary, as there is no central database of Steiner early childhood educators' email addresses to drawn on.

Translations and terminology

Translations

Potential participants needed to be sent an information sheet and a letter of invitation (Appendices A and B) explaining the research project. The working languages of IASWECE for communications are English and German, however, the working languages of its members are far more varied. Once the text of these two documents was approved in English by AUTEC, they, plus the questionnaires, were translated into the working languages of IASWECE members.

---

2 For clarification of how the word *staff* is used in this report, see the following subsection.

These languages are:

> *Brazilian Portuguese, Czech, Danish, Dutch, Estonian, Finnish, French, German, Hebrew, Hungarian, Italian, Japanese, Korean, Lithuanian, Norwegian, Polish, Romanian, Russian, Slovenian, Spanish, Swedish, Traditional Chinese, Ukrainian, and Vietnamese,*

making the questionnaires available in a total of 25 languages. The questionnaires were set up to automatically 'read' the preferred language of the browser in which they were opened, so each participant would have the text displayed in their language of choice. It was possible to change language at any stage during the completion of the questionnaires.

The question of language choice was important to address and is not without complexity. Some countries have more than one official language and it is reasonable for participants to expect material to be available in the official languages of the countries where they work, whether that be in te reo Māori (New Zealand), Irish or Afrikaans. However, while some countries have only one additional official language, South Africa has 11 official languages, India 23, and Mexico has no official language but rather 68 acknowledged languages all of equal status. Providing translations into all these was beyond the scope of the project. It was decided that if individual countries wished to translate the documentation into additional languages this would be fully supported, although in the end no further translations were made.

Translations were made using Deepl and Google Translate online interfaces, then sent to native speakers for checking and correction before being entered into the questionnaire software or sent to participants.

Terminology

Writing a report to be read in multiple countries needs to find a way to agree on terminology which varies by location and convention as well as by language. In Waldorf contexts, such words include kindergartner and kindergarten, early childhood educator, teacher, early years teacher, play group, assistant, administrator and trainer among others. Decisions need to be made which leave the text understandable, clear, and accurate. The following terms are used throughout this report:

> *Educator: The person who holds responsibility for a group of children aged 0–7 is here called an educator. In different countries this is termed a kindergartner, early years educator, early childhood teacher or similar. The term kindergartner is avoided on this occasion as in the United States and possibly other places kindergartner indicates a child who attends a kindergarten.*

Kindergarten: An early childhood centre or setting, early childhood program, home-based care, play group and similar are here termed a kindergarten. In Waldorf terms, this is most frequently a group of mixed ages, 4–6, but in the context of this report it references a group of children aged from birth to school entrance. Early childhood setting is also used on occasion in the report.

Assistant: Some, but not all, countries employ teaching assistants who also work with children but do not carry the same degree of responsibility as an educator.

Administrator: Those responsible for the running of the kindergarten, with no specific teaching functions are here called administrators.

Teacher educator: Those whose main job is educating early childhood educators-to-be or furthering the education of currently practising educators are called teacher educators (rather than trainers. See O'Neill, 1986, among others).

Staff: In this report, staff refers to those employed within Steiner early childhood settings and kindergartens. This group includes educators, assistants and administrators. It is not used in the North American context of office personnel and administrators but is inclusive of both teaching and non-teaching personnel.

The terms Steiner education and Waldorf education are used interchangeably. They reference the same educational approach.

Data collection and analysis

The questionnaires were run on Qualtrics software, a leading online survey interface. The invitation letters included links to the questionnaires. These were sent out in the appropriate languages to kindergartens to be forwarded to their staff. Surveys displayed in the language of the operating system of the browser the questionnaire was opened in, so respondents could view it in their own language. It was possible to switch between languages if necessary.

Data was exported from Qualtrics in Excel format for analysis and graph making. Responses were translated into English as needed, to allow for thematic analysis, to isolate and identify recurring themes. This is a standard method for analysing qualitative data (Braun et al., 2018; Guest et al., 2012).

Funding

This study has been supported financially by the International Association for Steiner Waldorf Early Childhood Education (IASWECE), the Förderstiftung für Anthroposophische Medizin in Switzerland, the Waldorf Early Childhood Association of North America (WECAN) and Waekura New Zealand.

The researcher

Dr Neil Boland has a long background in Steiner education as a teacher at early childhood, primary and secondary levels. He works in the School of Education at Auckland University of Technology in New Zealand and is adjunct professor at the National Tsing Hua University in Taiwan. In 2020, he investigated the effects of lockdown on Steiner early childhood settings in New Zealand and Australia, writing three reports for the national early childhood bodies (2020a, 2020b; Boland & Mortlock, 2020).

Timeframe

The questionnaires were open for the month of September 2022.

Dissemination

This report can be downloaded from the IASWECE website, along with a summary report available in multiple languages.

Potential Benefits

There are various benefits foreseen from this research project.

It is hoped that IASWECE will gain an overview of the circumstances of the international Steiner early childhood movement after nearly three years of severe disruption. This will help identify needs and challenges, assist with planning, budget distribution, and next steps to help support its members. It is also possible that this study will identify and indicate topics for further research to inquire into educator and child well-being, pedagogical approaches, challenges and so on. IASWECE represents early childhood bodies on six continents; as well as its forty member countries, there are around another 35 associate member countries.

For everyone involved in Steiner early childhood education, this report provides data on a range of factors which can extend and balance personal (usually local/national) experiences, and anecdotes about situations elsewhere. It gives a data-based overview of educator experiences on a global scale. Drilling down into this data allows for national responses to be collated and presented in a similar fashion, although this report can only do this to a limited extent due to limitations of scope. It makes feasible future comparisons between and among countries or between groups of individuals with different roles within organisation (for instance, experiences of assistants or administrators compared to those of educators). Using the information from the Blavatnik School of Government in Oxford, responses are able to be correlated with lockdown stringency and other factors to see if there are evident correlations which can be further investigated.

The Steiner educational approach is strongly relational (Nicol & Taplin, 2017). The qualitative questions inquiring into innovative and lasting changes to practice are of interest to educators generally. Literature on the consequences of the pandemic on children is still emerging. Because of the global distribution of Steiner settings, the possibilities which this study offers of international comparisons of multiple factors is unusual. There is to date no study which looks at how Covid has affected pedagogy in 'alternative' or holistic early childhood facilities or the well-being of their staff, students and families.

Participants

One of the guiding ideas behind the project was that everyone working in Steiner early childhood in IASWECE member countries would have equal opportunity to have their voices heard – assistants, early childhood educators, administrators, and teacher educators alike. This is the first time which something of this sort has been attempted by the Steiner early childhood movement.

In total, there were 1072 responses received to the first questionnaire and 308 to the second.

Table 1 Responses by continent

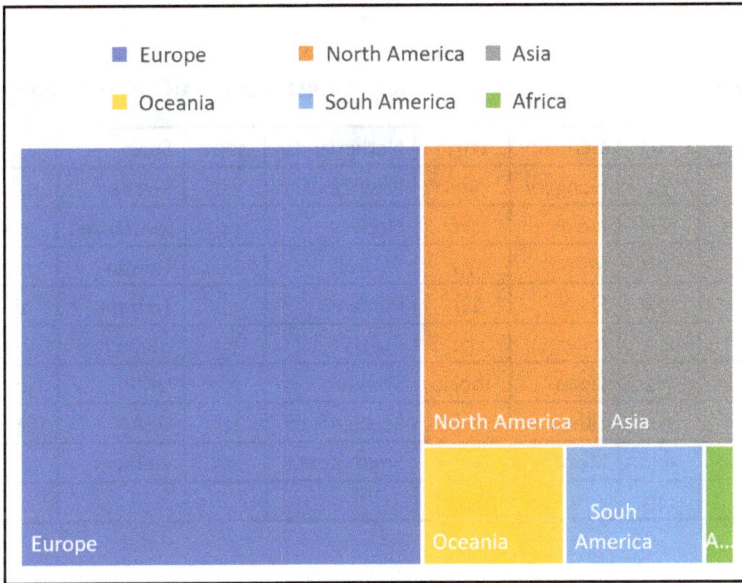

Table 1 shows the number of responses to the first questionnaire by continent as a ratio of the whole. Just over half of all responses (55%) came from Europe, as shown above, although European member countries make up some 75% of the total number of Waldorf kindergartens (i.e., responses were received at a higher rate from non-European countries).

Breaking this down by country, Table 2 shows the varying levels of engagement.

Table 2 Number of responses by country (Questionnaire 1|Questionnaire 2)

Australia	27|9	Germany	171|39	Netherlands	30|11	Spain	13|3
Austria	7|2	Hungary	33|8	New Zealand	35|15	Sweden	15|3
Belgium	28|8	India	7|6	Norway	44|2	Switzerland	22|5
Brazil	61|16	Ireland	7|2	Poland	22|11	Taiwan	16|1
Canada	19|8	Israel	14|5	Romania	37|16	Tanzania	1|1
Czechia	15|4	Italy	5|1	Russia	7|2	Ukraine	5|2
Denmark	9|2	Japan	100|36	Slovenia	15|7	UK	30|7
Estonia	11|1	Lithuania	10|2	South Africa	12|5	USA	164|43
Finland	30|8	Mexico	12|4	South Korea	5|5	Vietnam	4|2
France	14|3						

Table 3 expresses the same number visually, showing which countries submitted the most responses overall.

Table 3 Number of replies received by country

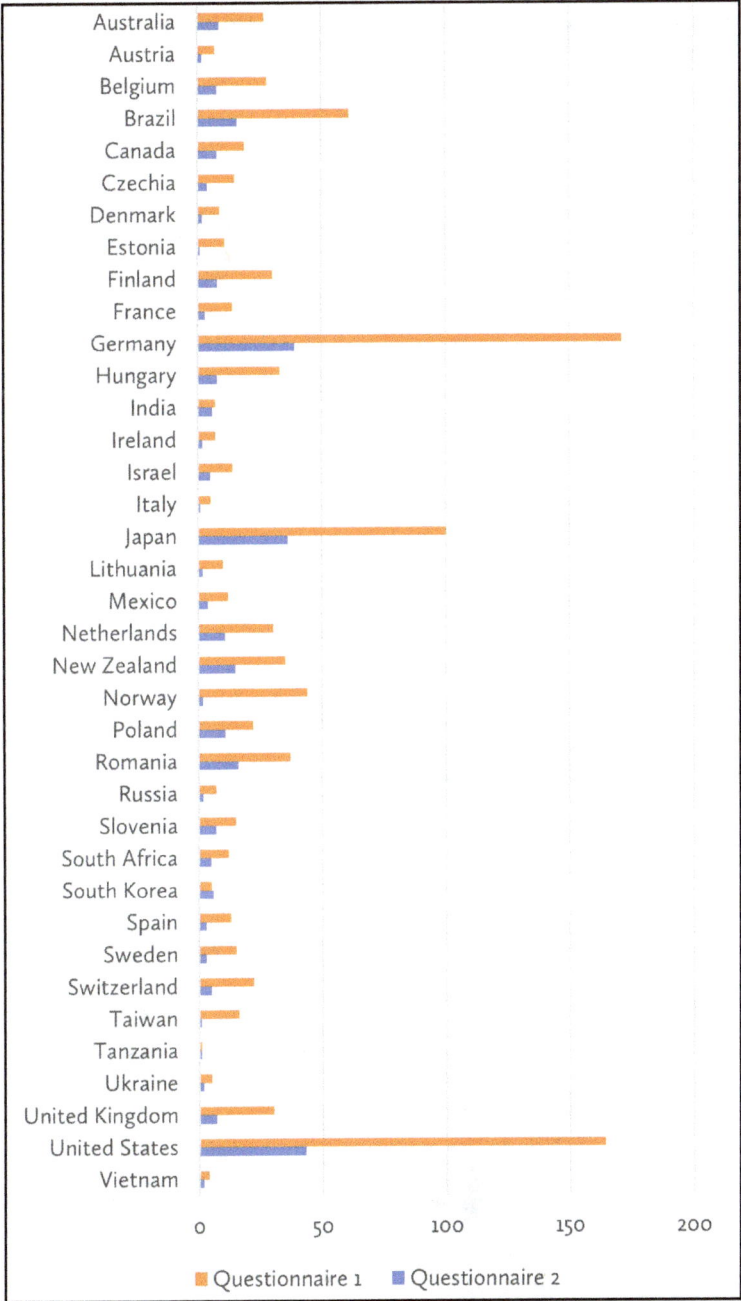

Table 3, however, does not take into account the wide difference in the number of kindergartens per country. For instance, the current edition of the *Waldorf World List* (Freunde der Erziehungskunst Rudolf Steiners, 2022) shows that, while Germany has 591 kindergartens, Tanzania has one.

Table 4 illustrates the ratio of responses per kindergarten in each member country and gives a more nuanced picture of engagement with the surveys.

Table 4 Ratio of responses per kindergarten

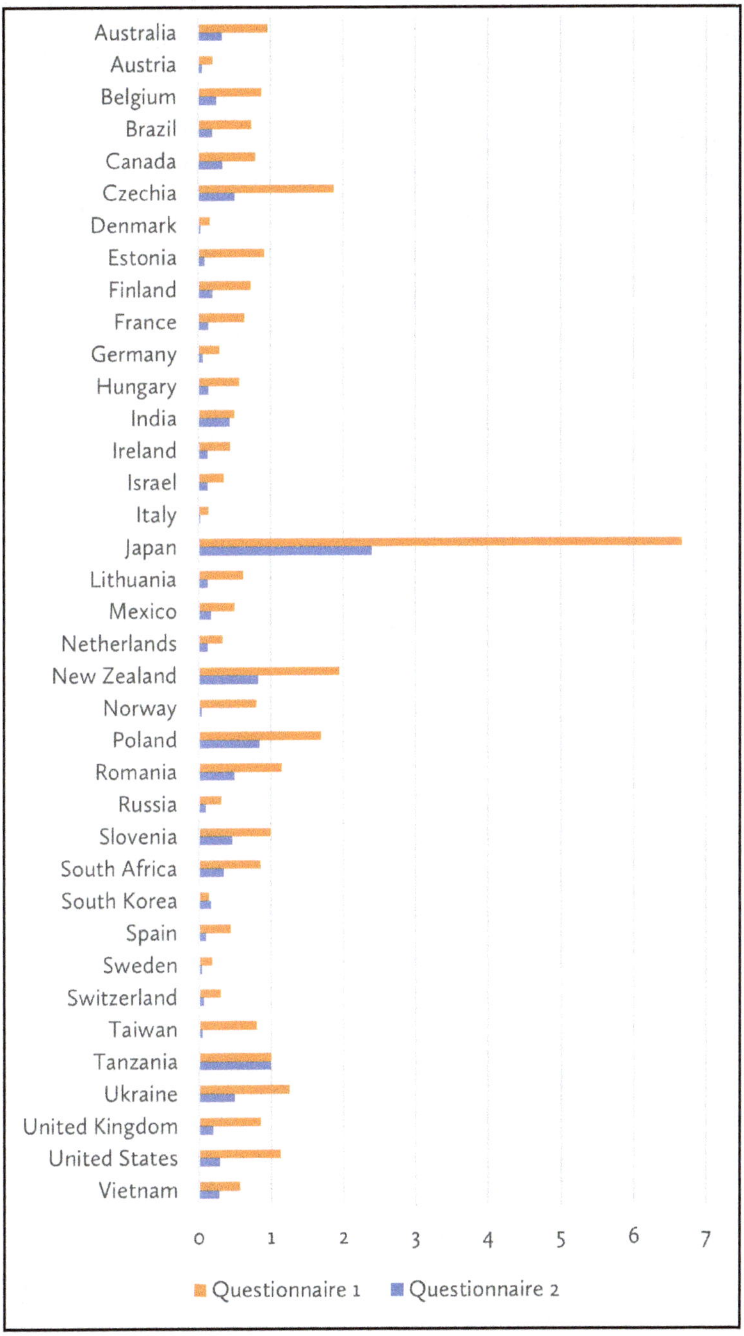

Australia
Austria
Belgium
Brazil
Canada
Czechia
Denmark
Estonia
Finland
France
Germany
Hungary
India
Ireland
Israel
Italy
Japan
Lithuania
Mexico
Netherlands
New Zealand
Norway
Poland
Romania
Russia
Slovenia
South Africa
South Korea
Spain
Sweden
Switzerland
Taiwan
Tanzania
Ukraine
United Kingdom
United States
Vietnam
0 1 2 3 4 5 6 7
Questionnaire 1
Questionnaire 2

The stand-out feature of this graph is the response from Japanese colleagues to the questionnaires. An average of almost seven staff members per kindergarten completed the first questionnaire in Japan (100 replies from 15 kindergartens) and over two for the second (36 responses from 15 kindergartens). This is by far the highest of any country. Particular mention should also be made of educators in Ukraine who, despite the situation in their country, found time and made the effort to complete the survey at a higher rate than in many other countries where daily and professional circumstances are much less challenging. Especial thanks to the respondents in these two countries.

Participants' roles

Table 5 What is your main professional role?

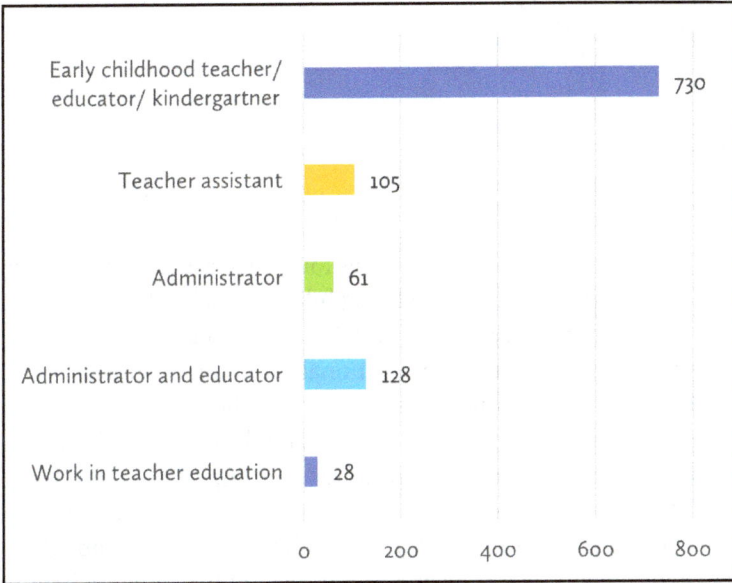

As expected, the large majority of respondents work as early childhood educators, with smaller numbers having other main roles. Analyses below show how individuals with different responsibilities have experienced the pandemic period differently.

No additional personal information was sought from participants (for instance regarding age, gender, length of time working in Steiner settings, level of education, full-time, part-time, nature of the early childhood setting, or similar). Future projects will be able to inquire more deeply into participant characteristics.

Additional responses

In addition to replies from IASWECE member countries, there were others (15) from non-members, viz. Colombia, Portugal, Greece, Turkey, Bulgaria and Albania. This report relates to IASWECE member countries, so these responses have been excluded from the analyses.

Context

The early childhood sector in general has long been asked to realise competing purposes. These range from being "glorified babysitters" (Osgood, 2021, p. 172), enabling parents and caregivers to go out to work to earn money and to support the local and national economies, while at the same time be providers of high-quality early childhood services which are associated with positive long-term learning and developmental outcomes for children. The early childhood workforce is strongly gendered (female), has low status within society, often receives poor pay and works in unfavourable conditions (Osgood, 2021). Depending on location and administrative requirements, early childhood settings not infrequently have to struggle with demands to "heighten professionalism" (Jones, 2020) (and conform to hegemonic framings of what constitutes "professional"), "raise standards" (Siraj et al., 2022), and buy into what are often neo-liberal educational agendas (Press et al., 2018; Roberts-Holmes & Moss, 2021; Wood, 2020). The sector has for decades been under-resourced and this has led to a higher-than-desired turnover of staff and staffing shortages (Kwon et al., 2020; Totenhagen et al., 2016). While these are characteristics of the sector as a whole, anecdotally, the situation in many Steiner Waldorf settings is not dissimilar. Research is needed to investigate the degree to which any of these characteristics apply to Steiner settings in different countries.

The above characteristics lead, predictably, to teacher strain, and it is acknowledged that, when educators are under strain, the education of those they care for is negatively impacted (Henry et al., 2021). There is an emerging body of literature which details how the pandemic and responses to it have (usually negatively) affected early childhood educators. The title of one of these, *My cup was empty* (McFarland et al., 2022) speaks to the experience of many. Worldwide, it has been reported that lockdown restrictions intensified situations already existing pre-pandemic (Flack et al., 2020; Gauthier et al., 2020; Noble, 2020). Those people in favourable living and working circumstances with sufficient financial backing found lockdowns by and large a positive experience, while those living under housing, social or financial stresses were more likely to find it negative. Similar effects have been widely reported in education as well (Haelermans et al., 2022) – students from disadvantaged backgrounds were much more likely to be negatively affected than those living in more favourable circumstances.

Challenges of researching an evolving situation

There are challenges researching the Covid-19 pandemic in that it continues to be an evolving situation (World Organisation for Early Childhood Education, 2020). Much of the world appears to have 'moved on' but new variants continue to emerge, and new waves move through different countries at different times. Normally, a research project draws from a body of literature which has become established over a number of years, with understandings gradually maturing as new viewpoints are explored and established. This is not the case with the Covid-19 pandemic. An increasing number of studies are being published and there are, no doubt, many more underway, but all the relevant literature has been written during the last three years and is subject to constant revision as new information becomes available. Peer-reviewed academic articles frequently take a long time to be printed, sometimes well over a year. This turnaround has only increased during the pandemic (Flaherty, 2022). For this reason, articles and reports from the media are a rich source of information when researching the current pandemic. Major reviews (Shergold et al., 2022) and overviews of existing literature (Jalongo, 2021) are only just beginning to emerge.

The following section gives main findings from both questionnaires.

Findings

Quantitative questions

This section details responses from over 1000 participants to a set of standard questions asking for single replies to questions on well-being, child development, enrolment and staffing and vaccine mandates. The results are given in graph format, which allows for them to be understood and interpreted visually as well as having some accompanying text. More detailed analysis is found in the qualitative section (page 58).

Q1 Well-being

The first section of Questionnaire 1 gathered quantitative data regarding perceived well-being compared to before the pandemic – well-being of children, of the participants, as well as of colleagues, families, and the societies in which the participants work. Each question offered seven options, ranging from *Much better* to *Much worse*. These are here presented in tabular format.

Your well-being as an educator

Table 6 Professional well-being

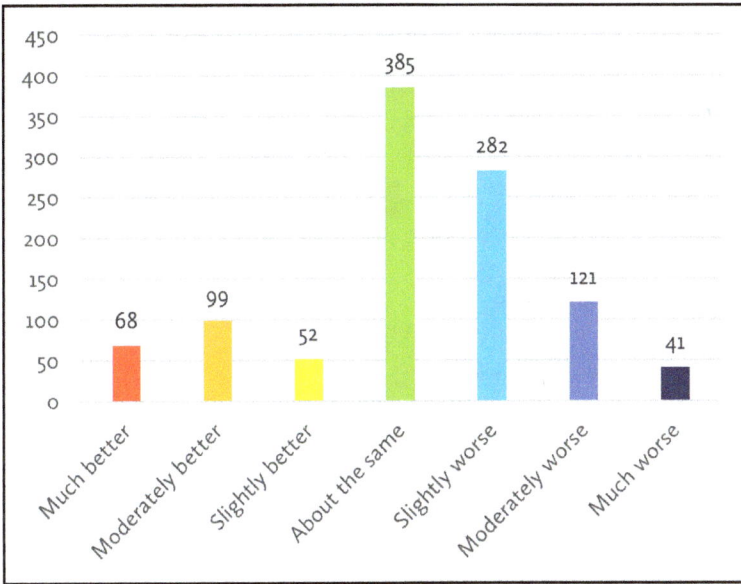

Table 6 indicates that around 21% of colleagues experience increased well-being since before the pandemic, for another 37% their well-being is largely the same, whereas the remaining 42% experience a decrease in professional well-being, with 4% (41 individuals) of the total reporting that it is much worse.

If this is looked at in more detail, it can be seen that well-being is experienced differently according to professional role. Table 7 below shows this according to percentage of responses by role (using all seven Likert options from *Much better* to *Much worse*). For educators, assistants, and administrators, while negative experiences outweighed positive ones, the greatest number of responses was that things were more or less the same. This is not the same for teacher educators, the greatest number of whom responded that their well-being was a little or moderately worse.

Table 7 By role as percentage

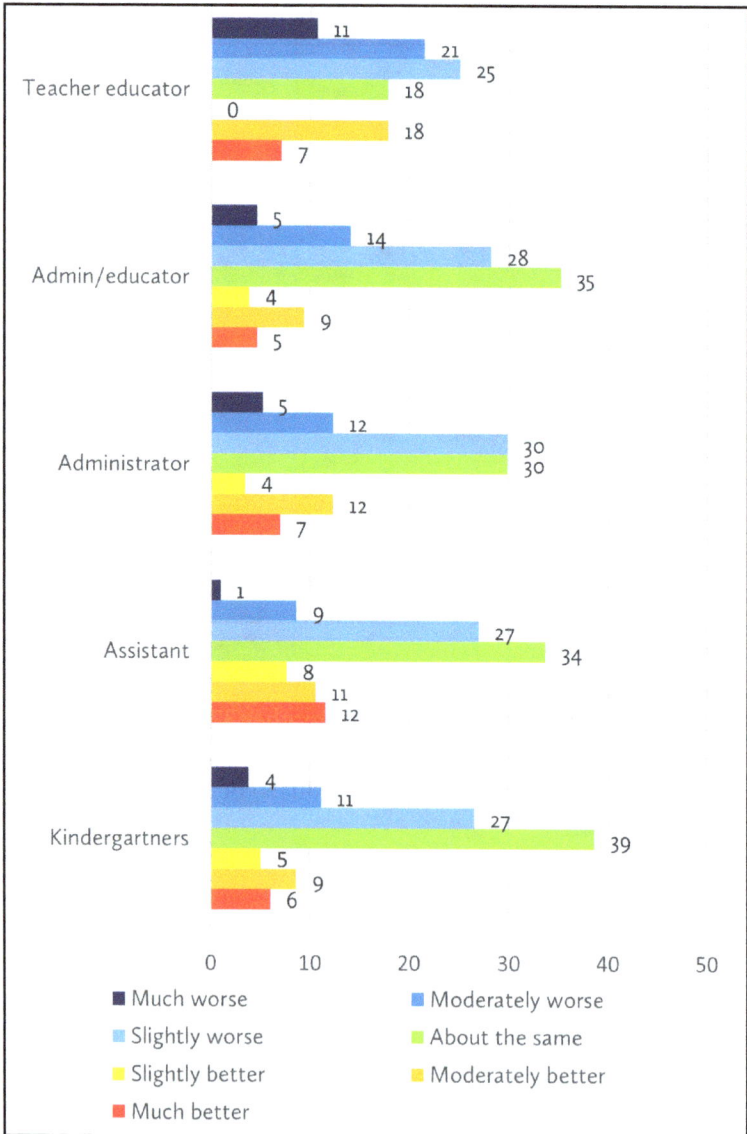

Table 8 shows this more simply, by compiling all the positive and all the negative ratings into one, to facilitate immediate comparison (in percentages).

Table 8 Professional well-being

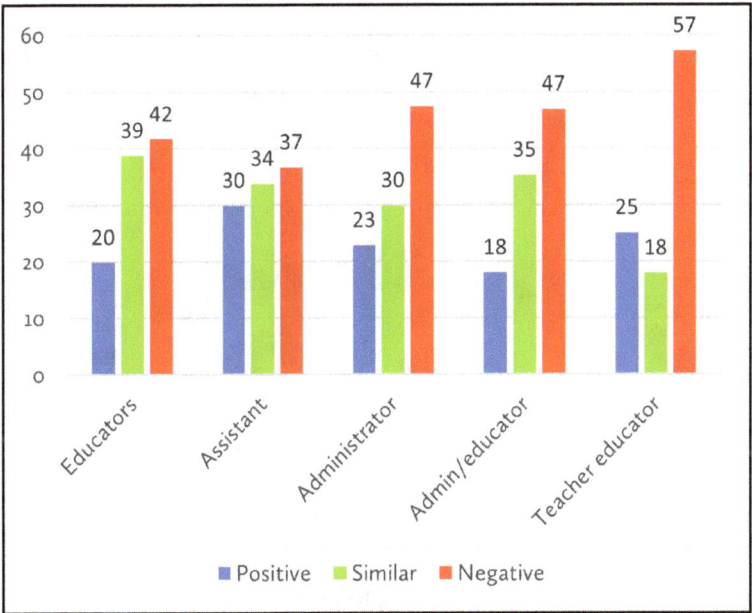

For every role, negative (red) experiences outweighed the other ratings. This was the most noticeable, however, for teacher educators. While 25% of teacher educators have experienced an improvement in well-being, a clear majority (57%) has experienced the opposite, with only 18% reporting that things are more or less the same.

This merits further exploration to see what has contributed to this deterioration of teacher educators' perceived well-being.

The well-being of children in your care

Table 9 The well-being of children in your care

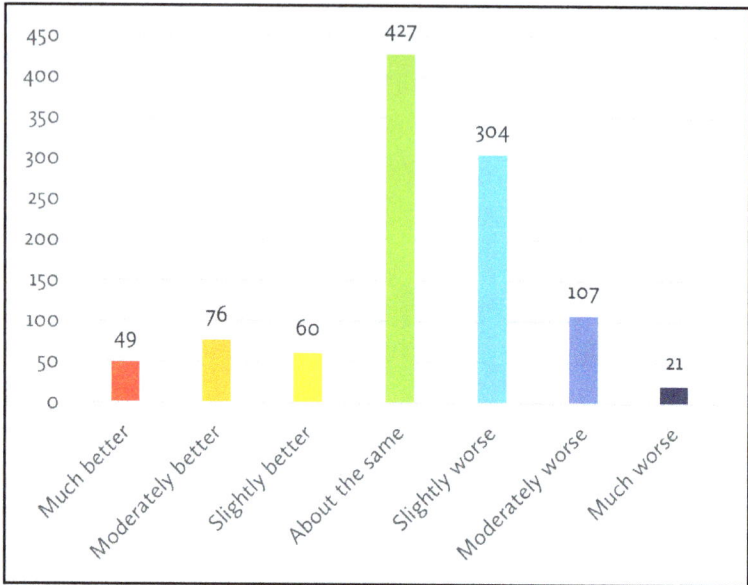

The overall outline of child well-being follows the self-reported well-being of staff in Table 8. 18% of responses indicate a positive change in child well-being, 41% about the same, and 41% a deterioration. However, greatly improved child well-being is reported at more than twice the rate as greatly lowered well-being. Comments from the second questionnaire around how the pandemic has affected children give detail to these statistics and are found later in this report.

The well-being of families

Table 10 The well-being of their families

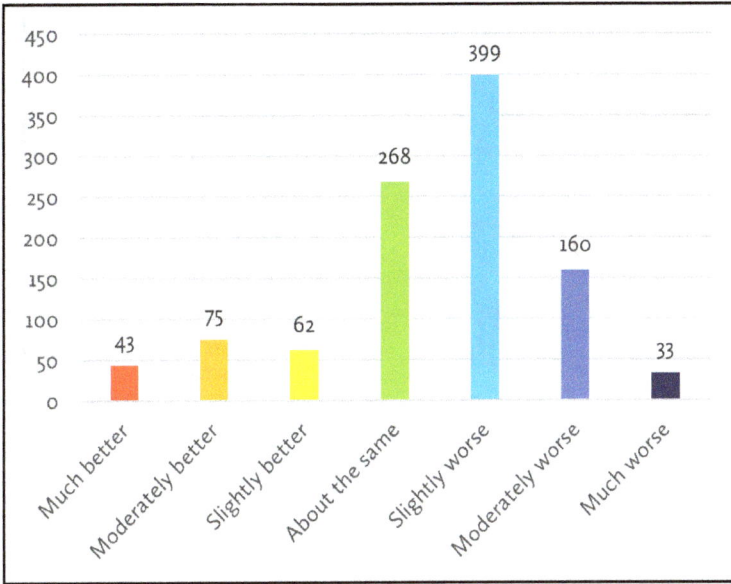

This is the first of four graphs which have a similar profile, where the largest number of responses indicates slightly worse well-being, rather than 'about the same' as in previous tables. Though there are few indications that family well-being is much worse, over half the responses are negative to some degree (54%) rather than positive (18%), indicating that the pandemic period has been negative to family life. While this may seem self-explanatory to some, it is in contrast to indications in some countries earlier on in the pandemic (Boland, 2020b; Greyling et al., 2021; Victoria University of Wellington, 2020) when families were spending more time with each other because of lockdowns and were reporting increased well-being due to this (involuntary) increase in family time—often high-quality family time. See page 76 seqq. for details.

The well-being of your colleagues

Table 11 The well-being of your colleagues

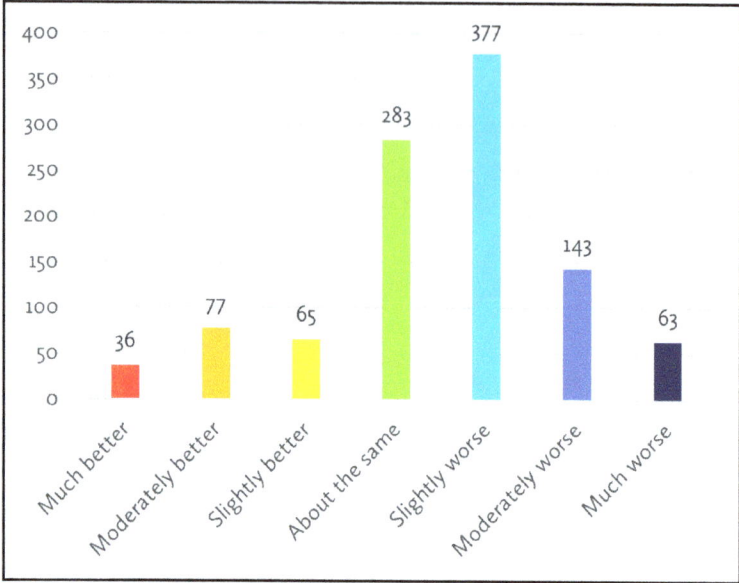

Table 11 shows a similar outline: 17% positive overall, 27% neutral, 56% negative overall when considering colleagues' well-being.

It is interesting to contrast this with Table 6, a self-assessment of professional well-being. The people represented by these two graphs are, essentially, one and the same. The difference is that in Table 6 they are self-reporting, whereas in Table 11 they are reporting about the well-being of others. Table 12 puts this graphically:

Table 12 Well-being comparison

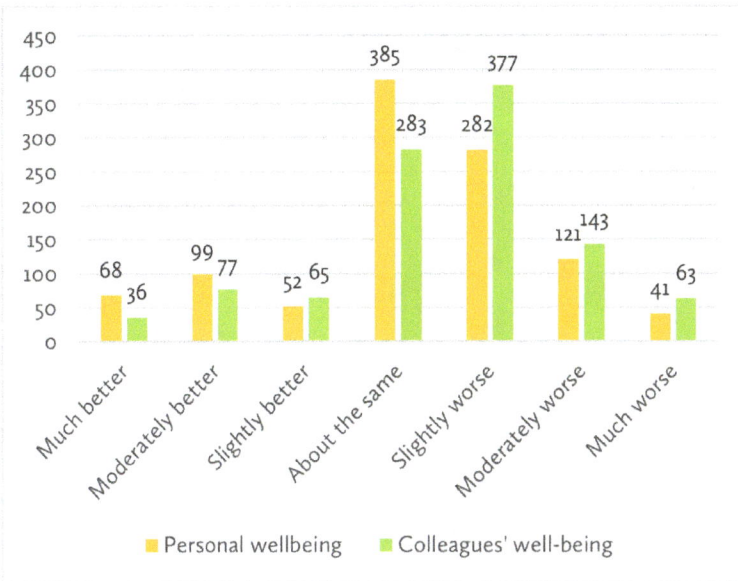

These two sets of data show that staff consistently rate their own well-being as higher than their perceptions of that of their colleagues. Reasons for this are unclear, however, there are several possibilities. One is that Waldorf early childhood professionals are slightly stoic, with an 'I'm all right', 'I'll just keep on going' attitude, making light of their own struggles, and more aware of others' challenges and needs. Another possibility could be that colleagues complaining about something or looking stressed or fatigued may lead others to assume that their well-being is affected, whereas it is not so much. It would be worthwhile to consider research into staff well-being in Steiner early childhood services to investigate this further.

The well-being of the parent community

Table 13 The well being of the parent community

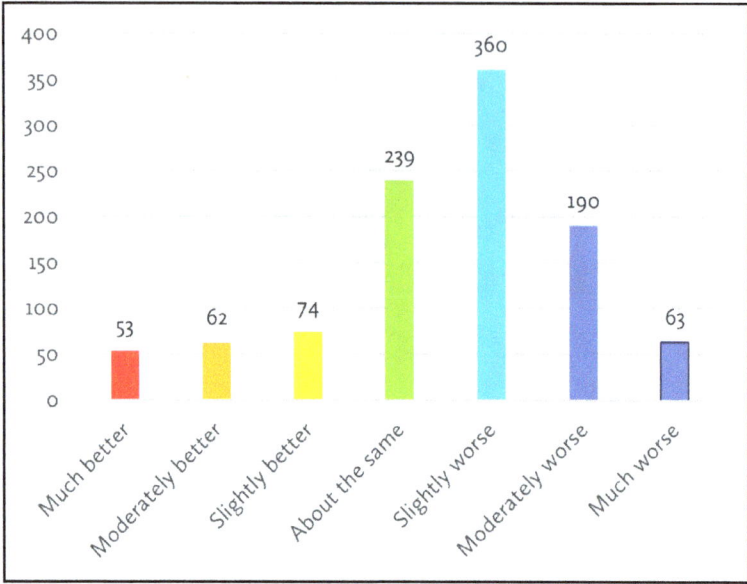

Parental community well-being follows the same general outline, 18% positive, 23% neutral and 59% negative. Pages 76 seqq. give detail on ways in which parents and communities have been affected by the pandemic.

The well-being of the society you live in

Table 14 The well-being of the society you live in

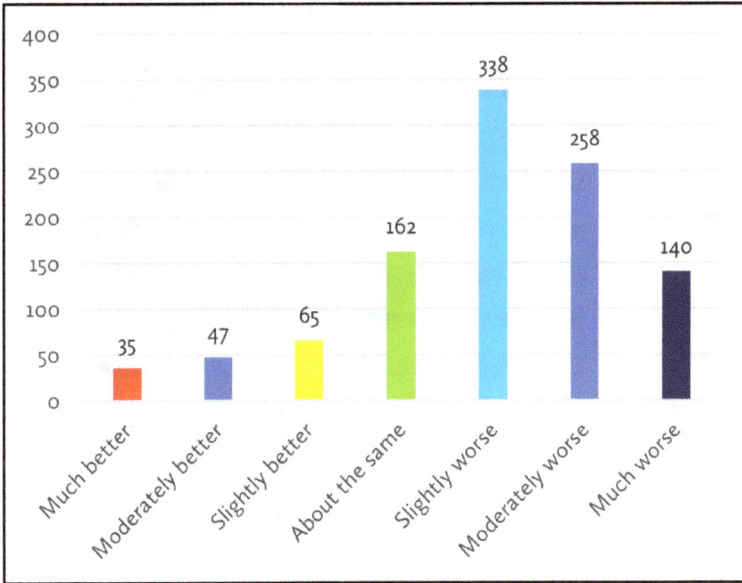

This question was included as approaches to the Covid pandemic have varied greatly between countries and there have been numerous news reports about the pressures which the pandemic has put on civil society in manifold ways (Bernardi & Gotlib, 2022; Ejsing & Denman, 2022; Farina & Lavazza, 2021; Shergold et al., 2022; Viola & Nunes, 2022). At first glance, this appears to be the most negative of this series of graphs. It has the fewest respondents indicating that things are more or less the same (16%), and a larger number indicating that the well-being of their societies is worse than before (70%) rather than better (14%). This reflects all that has happened over this period, including the increased polarisation of opinion found in many countries, increased inequality, added hardship for many, dissatisfaction with government responses and actions (and inactions), and so on.

Looking at countries with greater numbers of responses (25 or more), it is possible to see how this is reflected on a national basis.

Table 15 Well-being of societies as percentage of responses

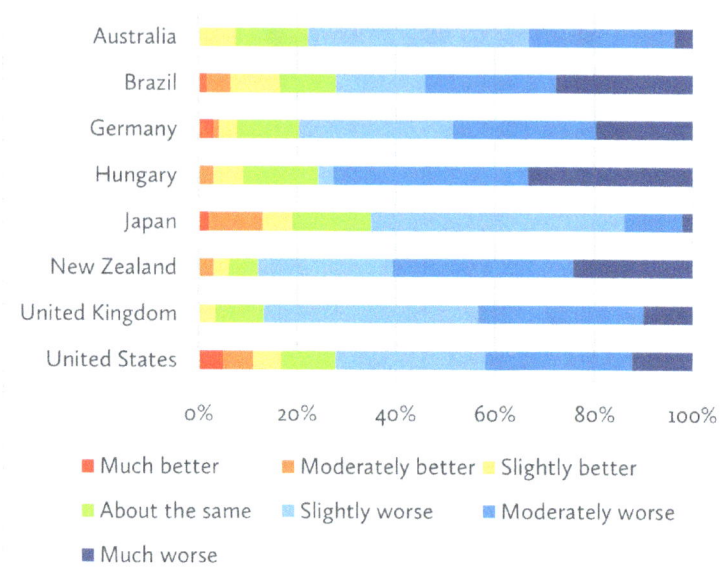

Warmer colours indicate increased societal well-being, cooler colours decreased societal well-being. What is immediately apparent is that, overall, the well-being of societies is reported as being significantly more negative than positive, yet within this, national differences are clearly observable. Exploring this by country by country is beyond the scope of this report, but it is worthwhile commenting on responses from New Zealand as it stands out here.

Of the 33 responses from New Zealand to this question, 6% said that societal well-being was better than before the pandemic, 6% more or less the same, and a strong majority (88%) that it was worse to some degree. This is the most negative response of those received which is surprising as New Zealand has been frequently held up as the country which has had one of the 'best' responses to the pandemic out of all the countries surveyed (Farrer, 2020). New Zealand has had the lowest number of Covid-related deaths per million of any country surveyed except Japan (Hungary has the highest of the countries surveyed) (Oxford University Blavatnik School of Government, 2022), has not been affected by unemployment to the same degree as many others (WorldData.info, 2022), and, although it may be surprising to many in the country, has been locked down for shorter periods than comparable countries (Oxford University Blavatnik School of Government, 2022), especially outside of Auckland. In the first year of the pandemic, it was reported that the governmental response was received overwhelmingly positively by the New Zealand population, including up to August 2021 (Molyneux, 2021). A study of New Zealand Steiner educators in 2020 indicated that 93% of them viewed the first (very strict) lockdown as positive or very positive for children, families and educators alike (Boland & Mortlock, 2020). What changed between 2020 and 2022 was that Covid became widespread in the country for the first time (from March 2022), much later than in other countries, and a vaccination mandate was applied to all those who worked in education and other sectors. This formed a focal point for groups with grievances against governmental policies, resulting in several weeks of social unrest outside parliament buildings in Wellington. Though New Zealand has a healthy history of protests, the one in February 2022 was unusual (in New Zealand) for both its length and virulency (James et al., 2022). Data gathered from New Zealand will be analysed in more depth in a separate article.

Your own well-being

Table 16 Your own well-being

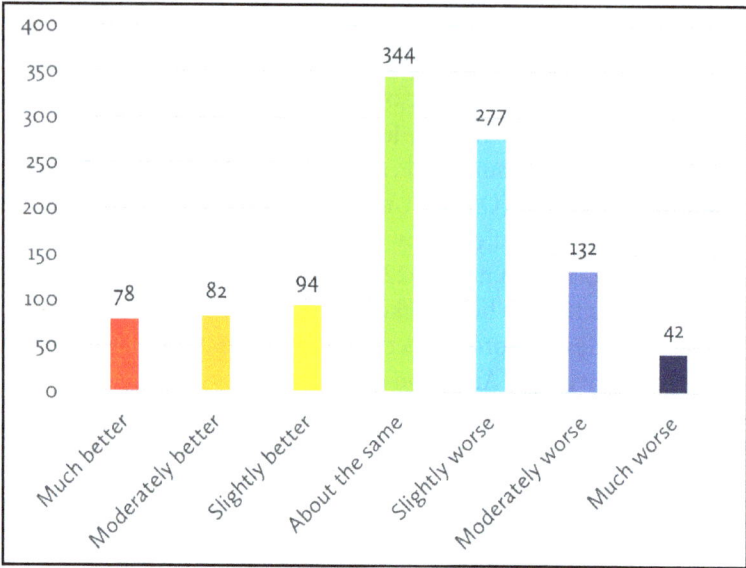

Table 16 looks at the self-reported well-being of respondents as individuals (rather than professionally). It largely mirrors how respondents reported their well-being, with some better, some worse. The two are compared in Table 17 below. Numerous quotations from individuals regarding their own well-being over this period are given in the Qualitative Questions section (from page 58).

Table 17 Private, professional well-being

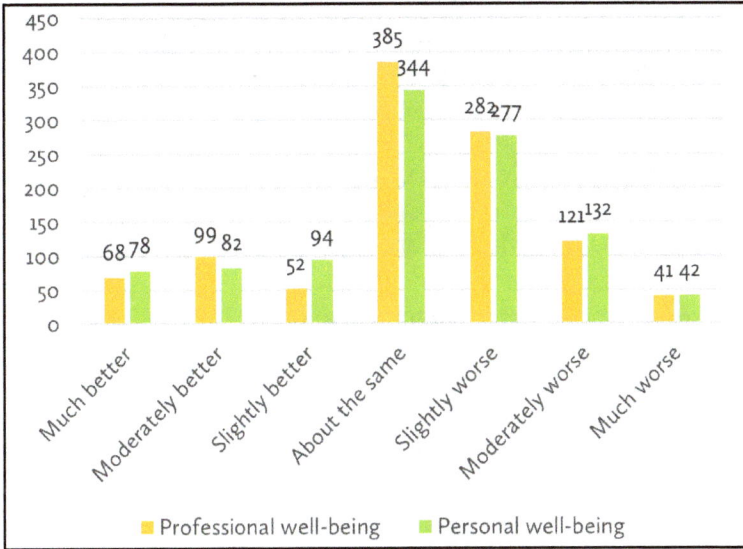

Chart legend: ■ Professional well-being ■ Personal well-being

Category	Professional well-being	Personal well-being
Much better	68	78
Moderately better	99	82
Slightly better	52	94
About the same	385	344
Slightly worse	282	277
Moderately worse	121	132
Much worse	41	42

Q2 Child development

The second section of the questionnaire looked at indicators of changes to child development and child behaviour compared to before the pandemic. These were regarding speech delay, movement delay, general vulnerability, anxiety attending kindergarten, separation anxiety, willingness to share with others, fear of groups and general anxiety. They were identified and chosen in consultation with IASWECE. Before presenting graphs on each of the eight topics, an overview is given to allow some sort of comparison to be made as to the strength of reported changes. This is done by giving values to the five choices offered for each question.

In answer to the questions "Compared to before the pandemic, how would you rate the incidence among children of the following:" The respective values given were:

Much less common	+2
A little less common	+1
More or less the same	0
A little more common	-1
Much more common	-2

For example, for Speech Delay:

Speech delay	# Responses	Value
Much less common	35	70 (= 35 x 2)
A little less common	60	60 (= 60 x 1)
More or less the same	519	0 (= 519 x 0)
A little more common	339	-339 (= 339 x -1)
Much more common	83	-166 (= 83 x -2)
Total / Overall value given		-375

Worked out in this way, Table 18, below, of all eight indicators shows a range of incidence. Overall, the picture is that children's development and anxiety levels have undoubtedly been negatively affected compared to before the pandemic period, although to different degrees. The charts which follow can only be indicative. Further research will be needed to explore what lies behind reported incidences of developmental change.

Table 18 Comparison chart of developmental indicators (minus numbers show negative responses)

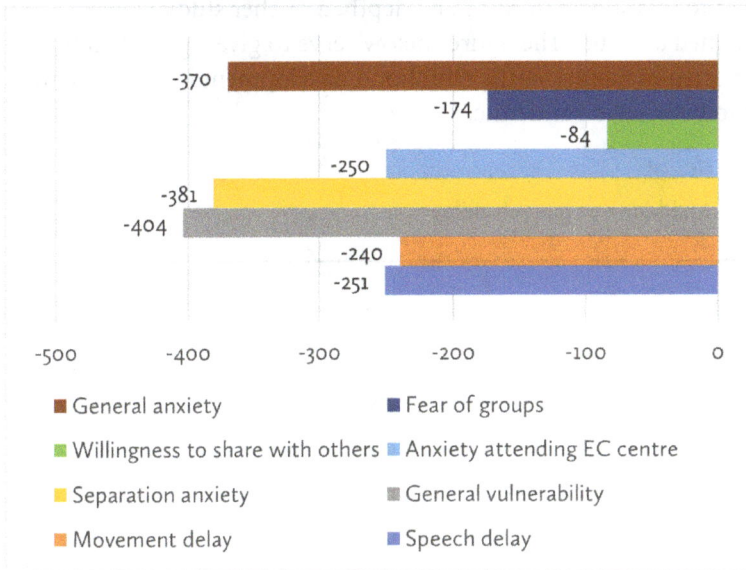

From Table 18 it can be seen that speech and movement delays are definitely present, and that general anxiety, including separation anxiety (being separated from parents/care givers), and vulnerability are the most prevalent changes. Anxiety attending kindergarten was reported at a lower level).

The graphs are here left to speak for themselves as they tell their own story. The numbers above each column indicate numbers of respondents. In order to investigate these in any depth, a further study would need to be designed and run. The figures below serve to give a global picture of the reported incidence of the childhood development indicators compared to before the pandemic.

Speech delay

Table 19 Incidence of speech delay

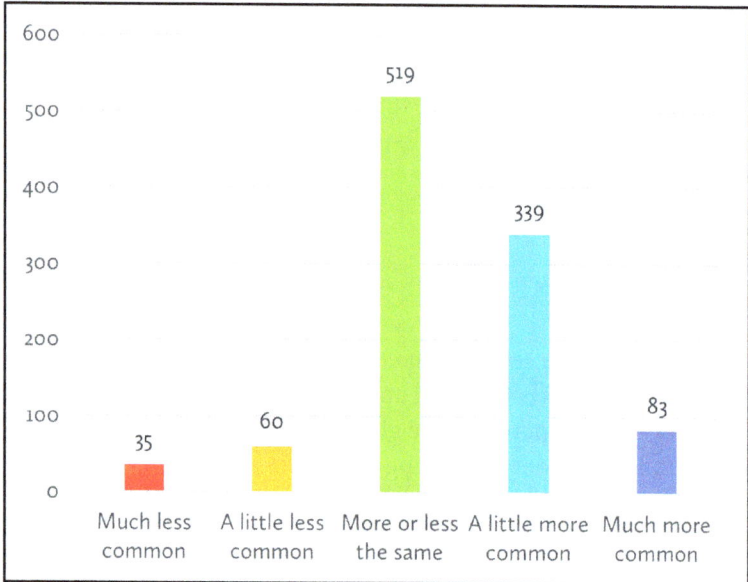

Movement delay

Table 20 Movement delay

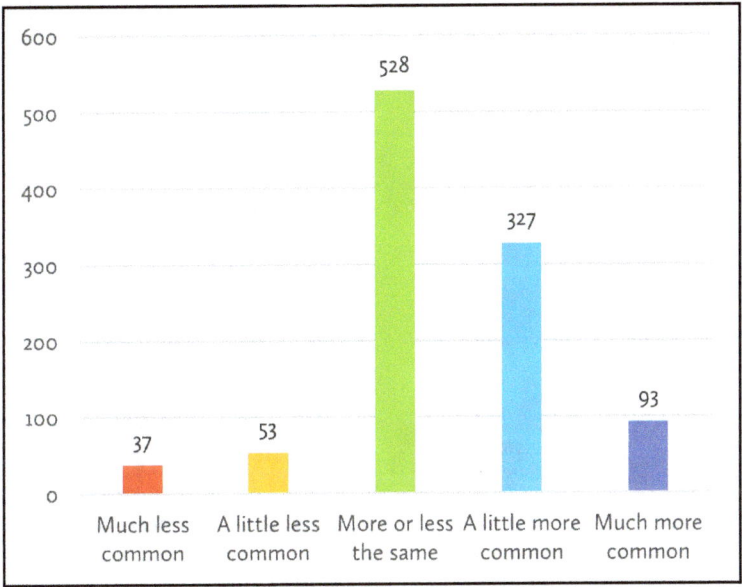

	Much less common	A little less common	More or less the same	A little more common	Much more common
Value	37	53	528	327	93

General vulnerability

Table 21 General vulnerability

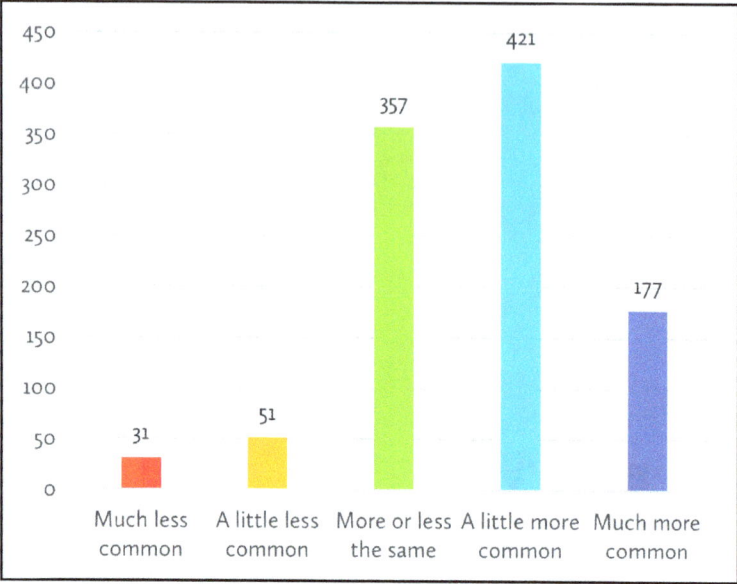

A general vulnerability was the most commonly reported change in children, compared to the period before the pandemic. Further research is needed to ascertain how this vulnerability manifests, but it is in line with existing studies (Zengin et al., 2021).

Anxiety attending kindergarten

Table 22 Anxiety coming to kindergarten

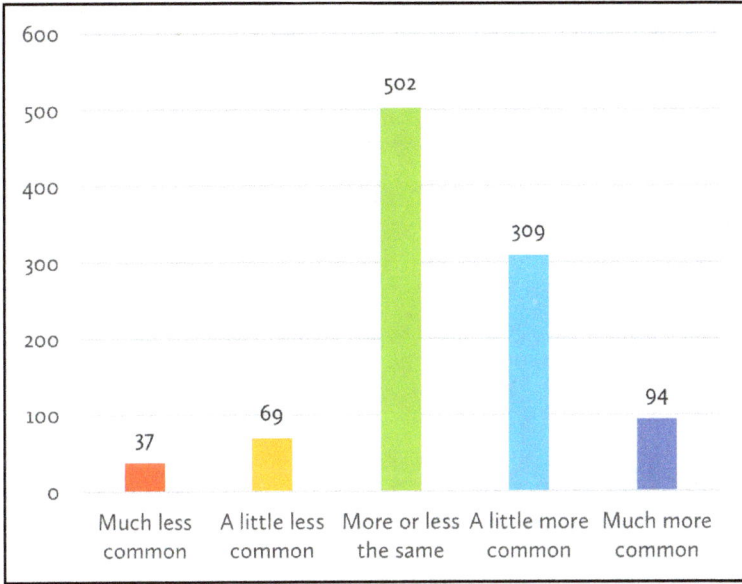

Bar chart values:
- Much less common: 37
- A little less common: 69
- More or less the same: 502
- A little more common: 309
- Much more common: 94

Separation anxiety

Table 23 Separation anxiety

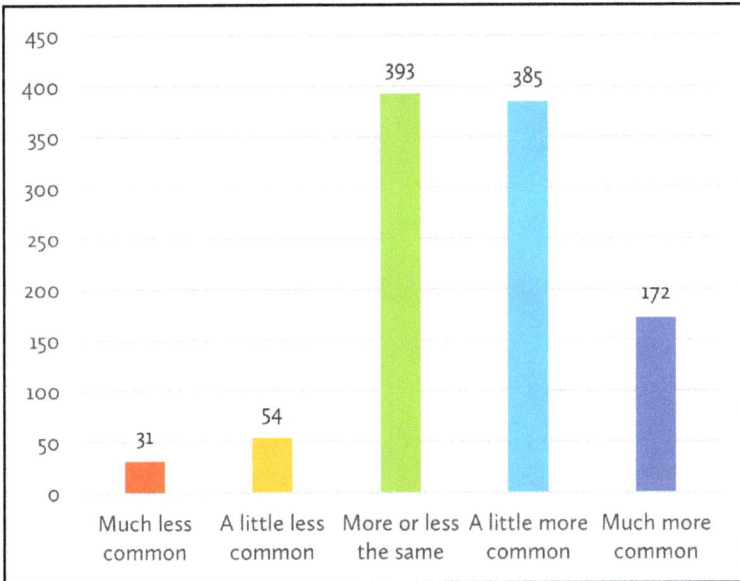

Bar chart values:
- Much less common: 31
- A little less common: 54
- More or less the same: 393
- A little more common: 385
- Much more common: 172

Willingness to share with others

Table 24 Willingness to share

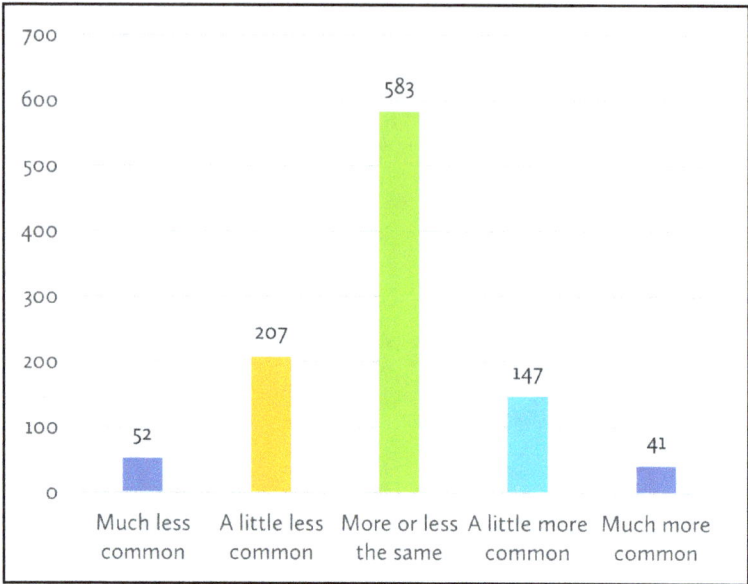

Of the eight questions asked in this section, willingness to share is noted as less common after the pandemic compared to before, although by a smaller margin (71 responses) than other factors.

Fear of groups

Table 25 Fear of groups

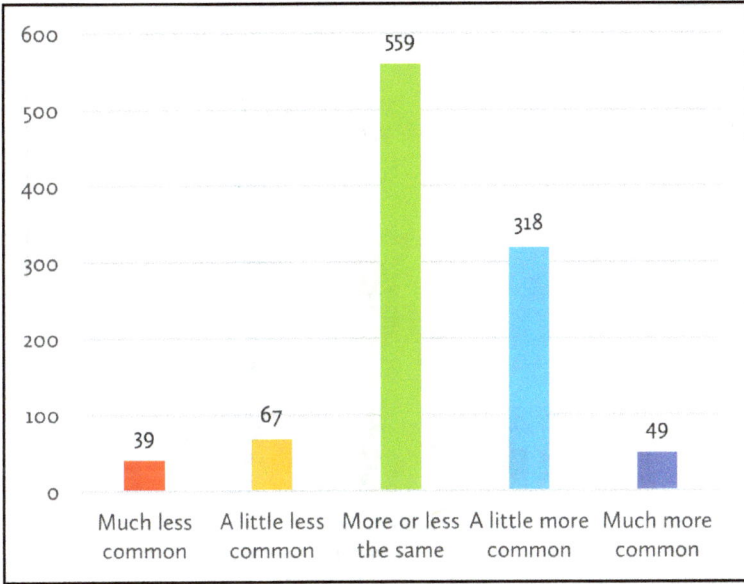

	Much less common	A little less common	More or less the same	A little more common	Much more common
Value	39	67	559	318	49

General anxiety

Table 26 General anxiety

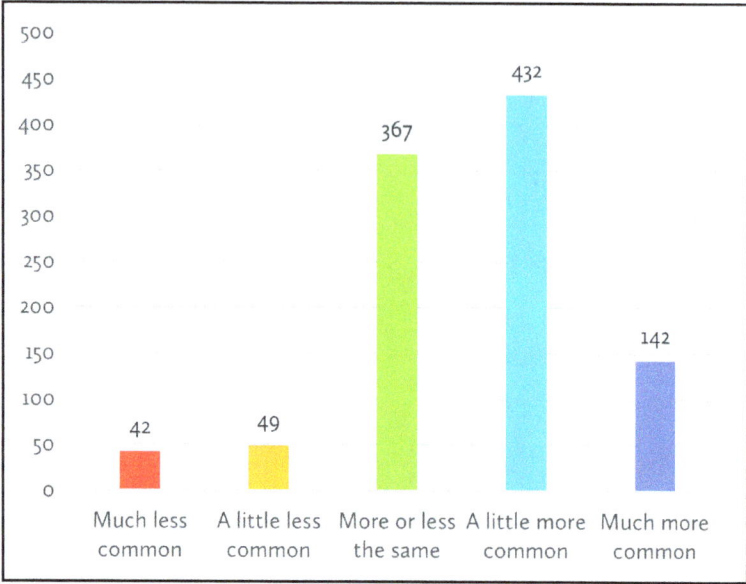

General anxiety is also reported as a significant symptom post-pandemic. It is worth commenting that anxiety in children does not feature strongly in responses to the qualitative questions in the second questionnaire. This could mean that it is not a significant issue in kindergartens overall, or because questions in this survey did not encourage further details regarding this. Again, it merits further investigation.

Q3 Enrolment and staffing

Questions around enrolment and staffing were included because anecdotally some kindergartens reported decreased numbers of both children attending regularly and children on the roll. There was also a higher-than-usual turnover of staff and difficulty finding suitable staff to fill vacant positions.

Compared to before the pandemic, there was lower enrolment:

Number of children on the roll

Table 27 Children on the roll

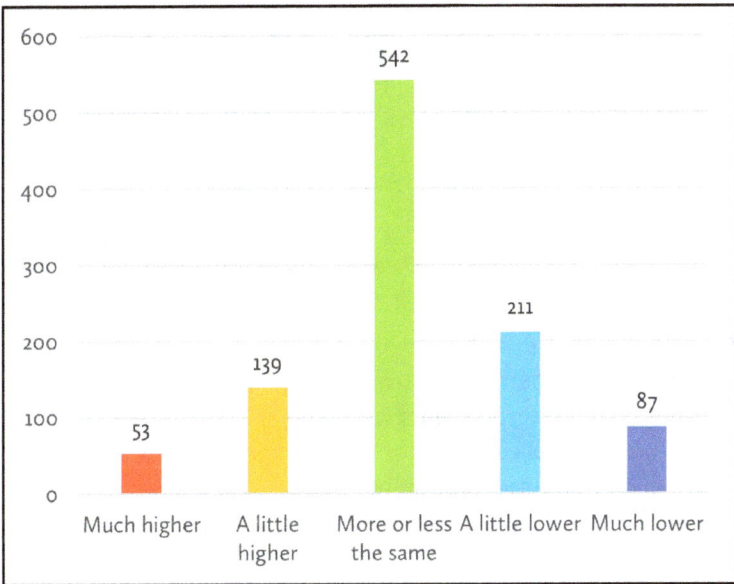

Overall responses indicated there is a decline in numbers of children on the roll with around 29% of replies showing a drop in enrolment, 8% a significant decrease. 19% of respondents indicated a growth in enrolments and 5% a strong growth. (The responses were collected in September, near the beginning of the school year in many countries in the northern hemisphere. This may or may not play a role.)

Number of children attending regularly

Table 28 Regular attendance

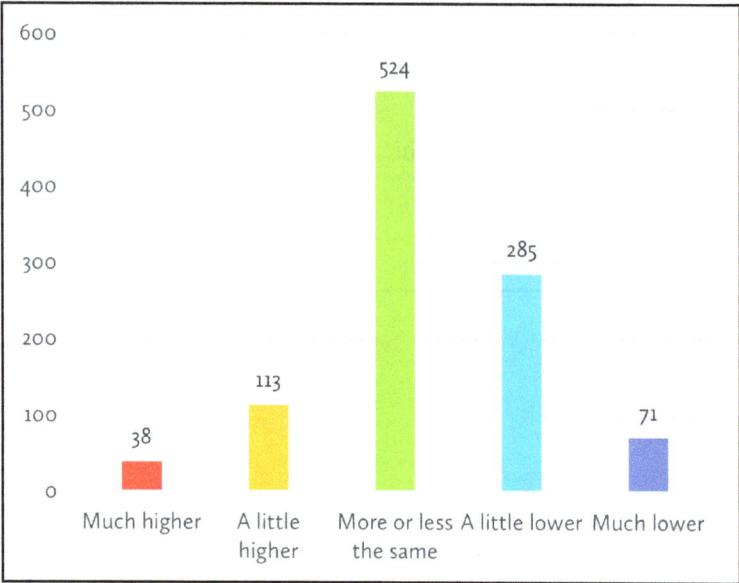

Regarding the numbers of children on the roll who attend regularly, around the same numbers of positive responses were given. However, there is an increase in respondents who report that children are attending less frequently. This could be for a range of factors. Covid-19 is still circulating in communities and there is a greater understanding that, if a child is unwell, or if a member of the household has Covid, they should not be sent to kindergarten. There is also a degree of anxiety among parents who keep their children home in situations in which they might formerly have sent them to kindergarten. This is explored in more detail below (see p. 69).

Staff turnover (compared to other periods)

Table 29 Staff turnover

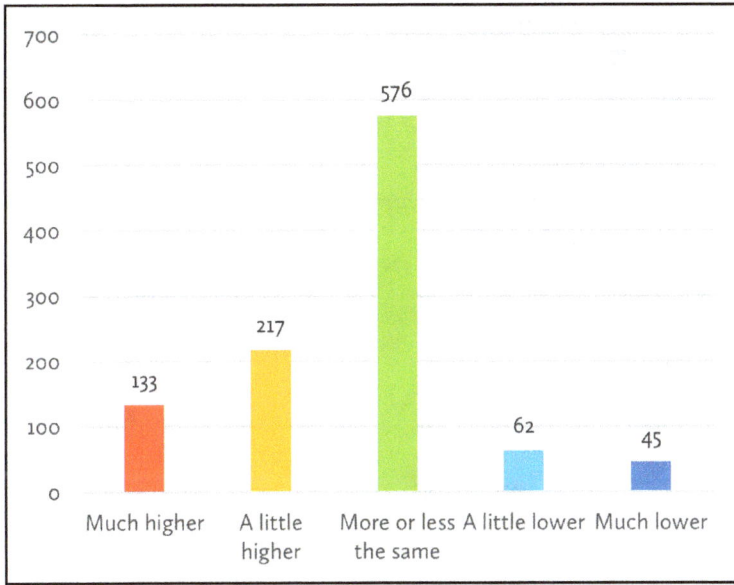

Increased staff turnover is frequently mentioned anecdotally as a consequence of the pandemic, as well as difficulty recruiting qualified staff. This graph gives some detail to these opinions. In some countries and states, the imposition of vaccination mandates led to a non-voluntary loss of experienced staff (see page 56) through non-compliance (Herbert et al., 2021; Will, 2021) who otherwise would have remained. Some of these people likely returned to work after the mandates were lifted, although not all. Numbers regarding this are not available.

There are few studies at the present time regarding the loss of teaching staff to vaccination mandates (see also p. 18 seqq.). A search of literature on the subject of mandates within the education sector speaks to a division between educators who feel supported or protected by vaccination and mask mandates and other health measures, and those who do not wish them to be applied. This is echoed in comments gathered on pages 68 and 85 among others. In her doctorate on teacher responses to the Covid-19 pandemic, Foord (2022) states that the majority of early childhood educators she interviewed (in a non-Steiner, US context) indicated support for enhanced health measures during the pandemic, including vaccination and mask mandates, if implemented consistently. "This had become a political issue. Teachers in my research recommended mandated vaccines as well as mask mandates. These would add another layer of protection for all students and staff" (Foord, p. 60). There is no current research into the opinions of Steiner teachers and educators in any sector (primary, secondary) on vaccination mandates.

The question of vaccinations and vaccination hesitancy is discussed below on page 77 seqq.

Inquiries and enrolments

Table 30 Inquiries and enrolments

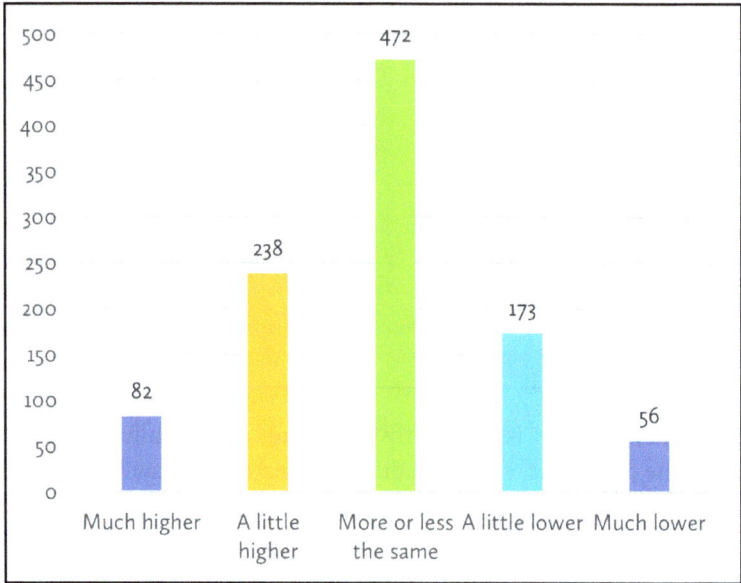

Inquiries and enrolments are reported at a higher level overall than before the pandemic. If this is looked at by country, for the eight countries with the highest number of responses, giving the values below to the same metric as for childhood development indicators (page 42),

Much higher	+2
A little higher	+1
More or less the same	0
A little lower	-1
Much lower	-2

we can see that the reported change in inquiries and enrolments is not uniform across all countries.

Table 31 shows the change in inquiries and enrolments by country given as a percentage of respondents.

Table 31 Change in rate of inquiries and enrolments

Australia	Brazil	Germany	Hungary	Japan	New Zealand	UK	USA
11%	43%	19%	28%	-3%	-38%	0%	26%

In most countries, inquiries and enrolments are up, most so in Brazil with a 43% increase. In the United Kingdom, there is no reported change, while in Japan, enrolments are very slightly down (-3%). However, in New Zealand 38% of respondents reported inquires and enrolments to be lower. Table 32 shows this graphically. (Having a value of 0%, the UK does not have a bar to represent it.)

Table 32 Inquiries and enrolments by country

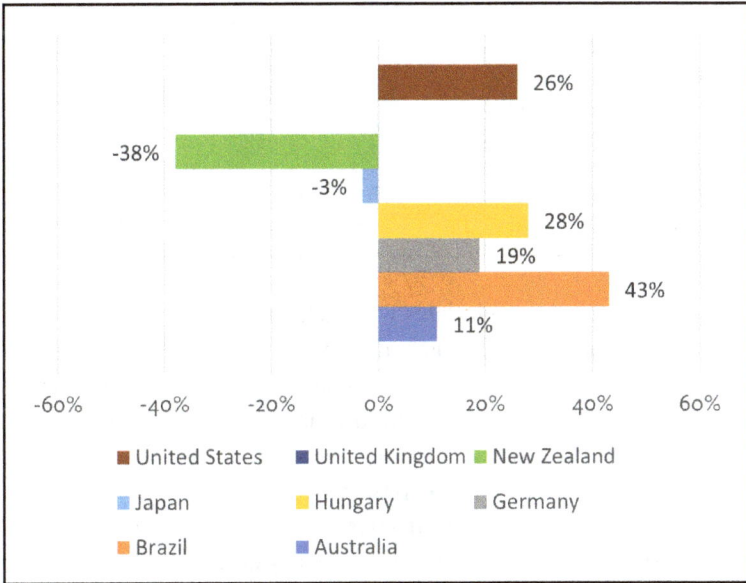

Q4 Vaccine mandates

Has your organisation been negatively affected by vaccine mandates?

Table 33 Perceived negative effects of vaccine mandates

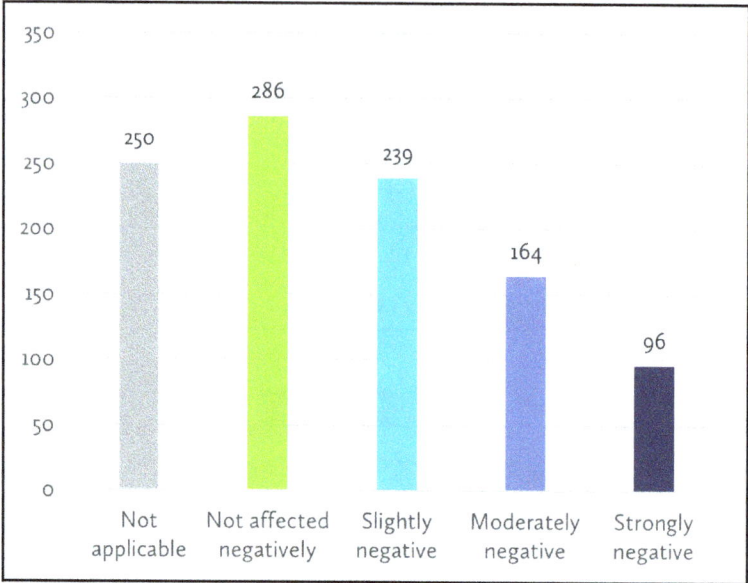

This question[1] on vaccine mandates was included in the questionnaire as Steiner kindergartens and schools had been in the news in some countries because of reported opposition from some parents and/or teachers to Covid-19 vaccinations and vaccination mandates (AFP, 2021; Mensch, 2021). The topic of vaccination and vaccination mandates has generated much discussion and heat over the past two years, with many people both inside and outside Waldorf communities holding strong views. This question was asked to gather information from early childhood staff about their experiences.

The statistics above give an overall picture. Of those to whom mandates apply/applied, over a third, 36%, were not negatively affected, around another third, 30%, slightly negatively, and the final third either moderately (21%) or strongly affected (12%). A lower number of answers were given to this question – a total of 622, out of just over 1000 respondents.

---

1 It was put in as a 'negative' question, which does not allow positive replies to be accepted (viz. my organisation has been positively affected by vaccine mandates). This was intentional, although it limits possible responses.

Table 34 Comparison by country

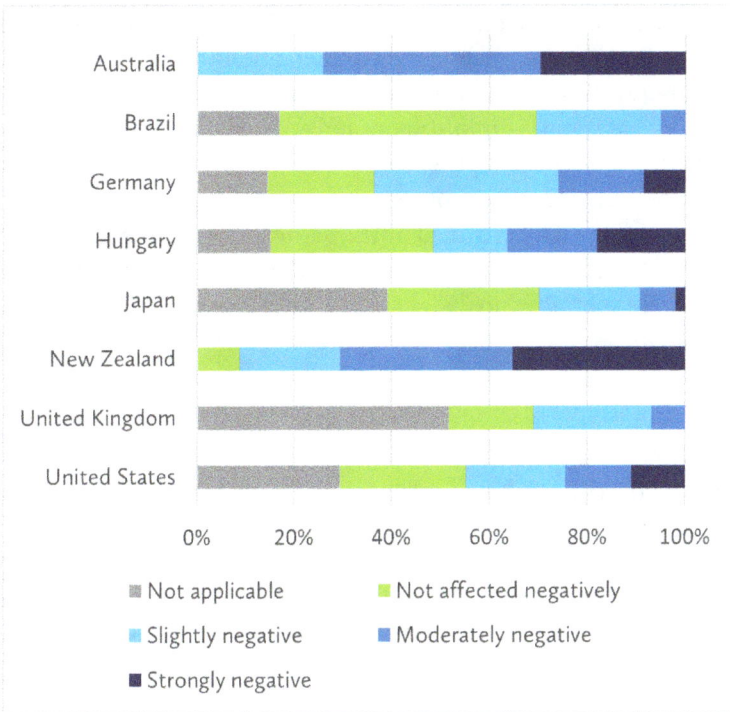

However, when looked at by country, responses to this question are highly differentiated, possibly more than any other. Table 34 breaks down the replies from the eight countries with the highest response rate. For instance, all Australian respondents indicated that vaccine mandates had affected them at least slightly negatively, with responses more or less evenly divided among slightly, moderately and strongly negative. New Zealand had the most strongly negative response overall, though 8% reported that they were not affected. In contrast, over two thirds of Brazilian respondents were not affected negatively. In the UK and Brazil, no respondents were strongly affected, whereas over 35% of New Zealand respondents reported that their institutions were.

Further responses on the topic of vaccinations can be found on page 77 seqq.

Qualitative questions

This section examines responses to the four qualitative questions asked in the second questionnaire, analysing them thematically to draw out topics which are frequently represented in replies. It allows the voices of individual educators, assistants, administrators and teacher educators to be heard. Due to the large volume of replies to each question (over 300), only a small sample can be included. What comes out in the responses reproduced here is the richness of the data provided by the participants. Further publications are necessary which can look more deeply at the themes identified.

Replies were submitted in 25 languages. These have all been translated into English for the purposes of this report.

Q1 Which of the changes you have made to your practice during the pandemic will you keep, and why?

From the responses given below it becomes clear that there is a wide range of views within the Waldorf early childhood movement as to which, if any, changes made should be retained as pandemic restrictions are lifted, or if the important thing is that former practices and habits should be resumed as they were. This results in tensions which are still being played out. A teacher educator in Canada expressed this succinctly.

> *These have been turbulent times for children, teachers, parents and communities. Many want things to stay the same, many like some of the changes. Much of the decision making has not been done with the children in mind. (Teacher educator, Canada)*

The question "Which of the changes you have made to your practice during the pandemic will you keep, and why?" was, to some, counter-intuitive, as how could educators want to keep changes which had been forced on them during the pandemic? In the words of a Spanish administrator, "*I find the question of what changes are going to be maintained strange.*"[2] Some educators indicated that no changes would be kept,

> *[The] changes...were cumbersome, illogical and hostile to children, parents and teachers. (Educator, Germany)*

> *The changes in our institution during the pandemic were mainly determined by the government. As far as possible, I will not keep any of these measures, as I do not see them as humane or appropriate for children. (Educator, Germany)*

---

2 Direct quotations from participants are printed in italic font. Small spelling corrections and other minor edits have been made for understandability.

I will not keep any of the forced practices that I had to do during the pandemic. What we should do was forced upon us, and it was something that I did not believe was the best for the children. (Educator, Norway)

or that "*No changes were made*" because of the pandemic (Educator, Belgium).

Such comments were in the minority – around 5% (16 replies). The large majority of the 306 respondents who answered this question reported on changes which had been adopted which they had found to be positive and which they are continuing. Analysing these replies indicated four emerging areas: improved management, the learning environment, health and hygiene, and improved training and education opportunities. Breaking them down by country is beyond the scope of this report, though it would yield interesting results. In each case, the country and role of each respondent is given.

Improved management

Responses here indicated that some changes made to the administrative work and communication with parents during the pandemic were perceived as positive and to be retained. The shift to the use of online apps such as Zoom and WhatsApp for communication and meetings was frequently mentioned. Some references were negative, but, more frequently, positive, stating that they had led to more effective and efficient communication and use of time (and, hence, a decrease in educators' workload). There were several instances where educators thought that using online tools to distribute information to parents helped ensure that it was more organised and consistent.

Some educators indicated that parent engagement had increased during the course of the pandemic, while some (viz. from United States, Brazil, Romania) added that online communication allowed them to build deeper relationships with the parents and their communities (10 replies). There was a perception that online staff meetings allowed for time to be managed better. Changes to management also included ideas for the better streamlining of roles, better use of space and simplifying various functions, helping reduce teacher workload overall. The use of online communication was also linked with ideas of self-care for the educators so they could spend more of their energies on their own well-being.

However, a large majority of educators indicated that increased reliance on digital technologies was not a positive move overall – they felt they were missing personal interaction and connection with parents. An educator in India asked for a "*hybrid model to work with parents*" to be adopted going forward.

Some representative comments:

> [Thanks to work we did during the pandemic], the whole management of the centre is more understandable to the parents. So, the pandemic actually made us improve the management of the school. (Administrator, Czechia)

> Meetings are held partly online, with fewer events and better time management as there are fewer appointments outside working hours. (Administrator, Germany)

> During the pandemic, we had to say goodbye to the big meeting with all 25 colleagues and are very happy to no longer have endless practical meetings where the majority of people sit around without really being involved. We have established a circle of group leaders in which all points concerning the kindergarten are addressed and worked on or it is decided in which group they should be worked on further. (Educator, Germany)

> Zoom parent conversations save time and allow all staff members to participate. (Educator, Israel)

> The splitting of larger groups of children into smaller groups during the week, we will continue. This has had a positive effect on the ability to give children more attention. (Educator, Norway)

> More digital education by sending videos and photos to parents and having the laptop with them at talks. (Educator, Netherlands)

> Sharing photos and short videos with parents [is a positive development]. The parents get a small glimpse into the classroom with pictures and that is appreciated. I do it less than during the period when parents were really not allowed in the classroom, but I hear it is nice for them. (Educator, Belgium)

Some noted the pandemic has initiated more efficient and effective ways of contacting parents (not for all contact, but for some things)

> During lockdowns, I sent the parent meeting form to parents a day in advance. This allowed them to prepare for the interview, and during the phone call we could then address what I had written, or they could add to it. This is something I will continue to do, as it gives more space/time to really engage with each other. (Educator, Netherlands)

> During the pandemic, we had to hold online parent meetings. Currently, we are conducting face-to-face meetings and online meetings at the same time. This is because parents who cannot face-to-face have a few more options through online meetings. (Educator, South Korea)

Learning Environment

Regarding the learning environment, a number of changes are reported to have been retained which were first established during the pandemic. Most frequently mentioned was increased time spent outdoors and a wider range of activities performed outdoors (all countries). Group sizes have been reduced in some places and there is less mixing between groups, indicated as a positive thing, which have led to a calmer teaching environment.

For some, festivals moved outside, took place without parents, and/or were reduced in scale and number. Several participants reported this to be a relief and a simplification of what was previously offered. Reducing the scale of festivals has led to a greater intimacy during them when they only involve children and educators.

The need to clean and disinfect toys during the pandemic led to some centres reducing the number of resources they had on offer for the children. Less sharing of resources as well as towels, glassware, etc. was also reported. This was found to be positive in many cases, leading to an increased sense of ownership and care of items by children.

Simplification

As well as in festivals, the theme of simplification came through strongly. This included the simplification of what is in the room, as well as encouraging children to use what they found outdoors for their play.

We simplified the menu of the snacks we provide; [before the pandemic] we gave the children too many choices and it was a good opportunity to look at it and simplify. We have much less left over now. (Educator, United Kingdom)

We spent more time with the children. I've learned not to run and that you can live more beautifully and fulfillingly with less stuff. (Assistant, Romania)

During the pandemic the children played with toys that could be disinfected daily. They did not play with dolls, cloths, knitted animals, etc. After the pandemic we provided them with fewer toys. I notice that they play more harmoniously, they cooperate better. (Educator, Romania)

More outdoor time, fewer toys (first for hygienic reasons, now for simplicity, imaginative play). (Educator, United States)

Slowing down the daily routine is good for everyone involved. (Educator, Germany)

We felt we were at our limit in many areas before the pandemic. The pandemic and the associated restrictions have slowed down our professional routine and shown us what really matters. This has been a very positive experience for us, the staff. (Educator, Germany)

Simplification. We spent so much more time outside with nature as our guide and inspiration in such a real hands-on way. I'd love to keep more of that, but my school and parents want more of the typical "Waldorf EC classroom" experience. It is not regarded right now that what we adapted to before is really also part of the "Waldorf EC classroom" experience. I saw so much build up in the children who came in person and navigated the social and inner worlds through being in nature. (Educator, United States)

Sharing of resources

The pandemic influenced the sharing of materials, resources and similar. Here, a South African educator explains how this has worked in practice.

Before the pandemic the crayons were used by all children. When we were allowed to go back to school, I made boxes for the children. Each child was able to recognize their name by the end of the year. At the beginning of this year, I started without the boxes, but soon saw the benefit and reintroduced them again. The children help with sharing the materials and they look at the names to place them on the table. Some children look for the name of their friend. The benefit is too that when a class activity takes place I can decide where each child is sitting. Therefore, an older and younger child sit next to each other in order to assist. This has been very helpful. (Educator, South Africa)

Parental access and involvement

All centres largely restricted parent entry into the premises for drop-off. This practice was reported to be beneficial across a range of countries, with centres reporting that children found it easier to overcome the sense of separation from their parents. Children adapted to activities in the kindergarten more smoothly if parents left the child at the gate, rather than on the grounds or in the kindergarten room. Of the educators who mentioned this, the large majority were sure that this practice would be continued. There was also, however, a thought that there was a need for *"parents to be involved in the morning transitioning period"* (Educator, Ireland). There was reduced inclusion of parents in the school activities. Festivals and events were limited to the children and educators which appeared to be more beneficial for the children to engage and enjoy. The number of community activities was reduced – some educators, however, adapted and held festivals and gathering outdoors so that parents were not disconnected from the centre's approach.

Dropping children off

Positive experiences in changes made to the dropping off of children were reported by several dozen respondents. This may be an instance where it took a significant event to alter what were established habits, in the end, possibly for the better.

> *The children are handed over in the morning in the garden. We keep this for pedagogical reasons. It is easier for the children to detach themselves, the children who are already playing are no longer interrupted by children coming in with their parent. (Administrator, Germany)*

> *The parents started to say goodbye to their children in the garden instead of coming into the Preschool. This worked really well so I decided to keep this practice up after the rules lifted. (Educator, Australia)*

> *During the pandemic, the parents said goodbye at the school gate and an assistant brought them through to the kindy garden and classroom to the teacher who waits to greet them. We will keep this in the future as it is easier for the assistant to deal with the separation between parent and child, leaving the teacher ready to receive the child happy to be in kindy. (Educator, Australia)*

> *We also changed the 'drop off' procedure, with parents dropping at the door. This worked well for separation anxiety. However, we feel it is important that parents participate more in the morning transitioning period, and so have returned to parents entering the building as before the pandemic. (Educator, Ireland)*

> *I am a teacher in a Waldorf Child Care. During pandemic, we couldn't allow parents inside the premises. I will keep this practice because children adjust much faster and are resilient. (Educator, Australia)*

> *We restricted parents entering into the indoor kindergarten space and have continued with this practice. It has been helpful to keep adult conversation out of the kindergarten, invariably parents begin to talk about adult concerns, and it disrupts play. Both the beginning and closing of our kindergarten days are so much more settled then pre covid. (Educator, New Zealand)*

> *I have a small Waldorf family childcare in my home. Since the pandemic we have had parents say goodbye from our porch – no more lingering – it has worked so well we will now do this forever. (Educator, United States)*

Despite my initial concerns, limiting the amount/frequency of parents in the room has created a calmer more secure kindergarten space. Going forward I would continue to limit the number of adults in the room. (Educator, New Zealand)

We have changed the way children are collected and dropped off at the end and beginning of the day, children are collected from the parents' cars, this has hugely changed the anxiety involved in children arriving each day. (Educator, New Zealand)

Before, parents could enter the classroom, but had a lot of difficulty leaving their child who might cry. This delayed the class a lot and did not help the child to separate. In addition, it could cause another child to cry again who had just managed to console himself and whose parent was unable to stay. There were situations of injustice and tension because the parent did not understand why he or she could not stay for part of the morning with us. By organising an arrival in the school entrance, the separation has become fair and easier. (Educator, France)

This has in turn led to an observable increase in independence on the part of children.

Parents wait for their children outside the nursery at the end of the day. There is no crowding in the changing room, children pay attention to what they are doing, they don't expect parents to dress them. (Educator, Hungary)

Children entered the school without parents and have become more independent as they hang their coats on the coat rack themselves etc. We think this independence is a great development. Parents no longer enter the school with us now. Ensures more peace and quiet. (Educator, Netherlands)

Festivals

Festivals are important moments in the life of any Waldorf kindergarten and form focal points for children, families and staff alike. When limits were placed on the size of groups which were allowed to meet, familiar festivals were either cancelled or found different forms. One of the strongest insights which came out of responses mentioning festivals was the benefits of simplification and celebrating festivals in-house with the children and educators only, though most centres report opening them up to parents again.

We have reduced our public festivities to one per calendar year and have also reflected on some other festivities. We have realised through the pandemic that we were overactive in some places and thus put ourselves and the children in unnecessarily stressful situations. We have focused more on the needs of the children again and have left the parents out of the equation somewhat – we now celebrate most festivities internally with the children in the groups without parents. So far, we have had very positive experiences with this – it is better for the children. They are less distracted, there is no need for a demonstration, the atmosphere can be held better, staff are less stressed and can concentrate completely on the children. (Educator, Germany)

We are very happy that at the moment we can celebrate all the festivals together with the parents again, because it has a very community-building effect and a good community is very important, especially for the self-governing kindergartens. In the case of the Advent Garden, we experienced that it was more beneficial for the children to experience it on Monday mornings, without parents, only in the circle of the kindergarten group. In this way, the children were completely in their usual rhythm and completely concentrated on what was happening. We are now really faced with the serious question of whether we should not continue with this emergency solution created by Corona. (Educator, Germany)

It was a relief to "do less" during the pandemic in terms of festivals and inviting parents to the setting but we will re-introduce that as it is important for parents. (Educator, United Kingdom)

Outdoors

Educators also emphasised the need to continue outdoor activities, as they were easier to manage than indoor activities which required resources and toys to be sanitised. The educators who mentioned it, unanimously encouraged this practice be maintained. While some educators felt online sessions with children could be helpful, allowed educators to look after their own well-being and become more familiar with digital tools, outdoor learning was greatly preferred. These ideas are also linked to themes of health and hygiene and improved training mentioned below. Changes in the learning environment made some educators more conscious of ideas of routine, rhythm, proximity and the developmental needs of the children, and question what had been done automatically as a matter or habit or tradition before the pandemic. Some Australian educators highlighted some aspects of a change in approach or attitude that was needed post-pandemic. "*I have become more involved in scaffolding children's play as their development of play skills has deteriorated. I provide more one-to-one reassurance and guidance as children seem more anxious*" (Educator, Australia). Another Australian teacher, however, felt that she was now "*more flexible and sensitive to children's moods*". Aspects such as smaller group sizes, fewer toys and equipment, more creative sensory stimulating activities, less structure, and free play were changes to the learning environment that the educators wanted to bring closer to the essential "hands-on way" of Waldorf education.

> *During the pandemic, everyone was out all day, except for a few children who slept in after lunch. This was positive in many ways and has been largely maintained. (Educator, Denmark)*

> *One important change that I made soon after the school reopened and that I still maintain today is to get out of the "recipe" – half the morning in the classroom, half the morning out of the classroom. I realized that the children needed to be outside, in nature, moving widely, breathing. (Educator, Brazil)*

> *Bringing and picking up the children via the garden. … Celebrate festivals in the garden or in the forest. (Educator, Austria)*

> *More free play. More exercise. More time in the forest. (Educator, Switzerland)*

> *Spending more time outside, my whole program shifted to 100% outside, the parents and children thrive in the outdoors (as do I). (Educator, Canada)*

> *Increased awareness of sense activity. Replace buckets or spades with coconut shells and sticks – for expending more energy and [increasing] sensory experiences. Longer walks in the parks – now thrice a week for an hour. Encouraging children to eat Indian herbs before entering the environment ("magic leaves that help keep your voice golden indoors") more varieties of fruit to eat at fruit break in larger chunks – to encourage chewing more and exploring different tastes and flavours – shorter morning circle with more movements – daily foot massages for some – less speaking to the children, more silent hand gestures – to encourage sensitivity to more non-verbal communication. (Educator, India)*

> *We try to walk barefoot on most outdoor trips. Walks in the parks. Apart from asking children for help for garden activities – we are making a more active effort to grow things /make compost. Sitting and ob-*

serving nature more rather than touching it as children did not know how to hold a worm for example. Active focus on cleaning indoors and outdoors. (Educator, India)

Health and hygiene

The emphasis on health and hygiene measures included the need to provide a healthier and cleaner environment for the children, as well as an opportunity for educators to focus on their own mental health. The health measures put in place were discussed largely in tandem with the increased use of outdoor space. Educators noted that activities such as walking, running, being in nature and the outdoors, engaging with elements of nature were health giving. Some stated it boosted children's immunity. Hygiene measures were discussed by many; aspects of hand-washing, distance, wearing masks, and cleaning surfaces were emphasised most strongly by educators in Japan and South Korea, countries which had a history of mask wearing before the pandemic. Educators in New Zealand, Mexico, Finland, Ukraine and Vietnam indicated that increased handwashing and closer monitoring of children's health were practices which would be continued. Educators in other countries chose to focus implicitly on health through ensuring activities are in nature and the outdoors. Some respondents included their own well-being while discussing aspects of health. Mention of less stress among educators through online communication was observed by a significant number of educators. Explicit mention of being able to *"take better care of myself"* and *"creating a better work life balance"* was mentioned by educators from Canada, while educators from Brazil and India talked about the opportunity for greater self-care which had arisen through the disruption caused by the pandemic and the need to continue it.

Hand hygiene

Positive changes which will be kept:

> *Ritualised hand washing before meals, some stricter hygiene measures, the daily cleaning of door handles and light switches. (Administrator, Germany)*

> *We have not kept any of the extreme protocols, however, a good relationship with cleanliness and tidiness is a healthy practice to maintain. (Educator, South Africa)*

> *1. Handy outdoor individual drink bottles instead of shared jug and continual washing. 2. Individual personal hand towels. 3. Thorough effective hand washing. 4. More regular door handle and toilet cleaning.*

5. More outdoor activities with families - in nature and the surrounding environment...the hygiene and individual cleaning regimes hold them in good stead for further independence. The outdoors communal activities were both 'fresher', enlivened, less restricted... at the same time we became more inventive to create intimate cosy reverent spaces in nature. (Educator, Australia)

Masks

The use of masks in early childhood settings has been controversial in many places, particularly that children's language acquisition may be affected by not being able to see the mouths of those around them.

The children spend the daytime without masks, but the caregivers wear masks and are constantly concerned about how this affects the physical and mental development required in early childhood, such as not being able to see the caregivers' facial expressions. (Educator, Japan)

Will being forced to wear a mask allow the important things to be nurtured? It is impossible to predict at the moment what impact it will have in later years. (Educator, Japan)

I have observed that measures such as wearing masks when working with the children make them more fearful. They have problems understanding me and are much more hesitant to come to me to address problems. (Educator, Germany)

We started an outdoor school because of Covid with no masks and no social distancing and intend to keep it that way because outdoor play and nature are very beneficial to the young child. (Educator, United States)

A different and insightful way of looking at this, arising from personal experience, was given by an educator from Japan.

In Japan, because it is required, [we wear masks]. At first, I wondered if not being able to see my mouth would have a decisive effect on children's development. I was concerned but, as far as I can experience, the children's whole body is a sensory organ and they do not learn words [just] by looking at people's mouths, nor do they feel the hearts and smiles of their caregivers [just by looking at them]. The reality, I feel, is that children receive love and words from their caregivers no differently, even if they are wearing a mask. [I feel] that the younger the child, the truer this is. (Educator, Japan)

The question of the effect the feelings of the teacher towards having to wear a mask have on the child was not brought up in the survey.

Relationship to reporting sick

A significant change which was reported to have occurred thanks to the pandemic is that people – children, parents and staff alike – are more conscious of the consequences of coming in sick and, instead, stay home and do not risk spreading the illness further. Early childhood facilities are traditionally hotbeds for colds and other ailments, and staff have to work with children who possibly should have been kept home. Similarly, it is not uncommon for staff themselves to come in when unwell so as to avoid needing to call in a relieving teacher and for other reasons. That new habits appear to be forming is to be welcomed for child and educator well-being alike.

> *Children stay home when they are sick now because it is no longer PC to come to work/school when we are not well. (Educator, United States)*

> *[We are] more vigilant about illness and to require parents to keep sick children home. Before the pandemic, we tolerated many ill students at school – spreading illness to peers and faculty. (Educator, United States)*

> *If you are sick, stay home, for both Staff and Children. This has been our most challenging and fruitful policy to enforce. Having more strict guidelines and follow through has benefited both adults and children. Our staff is less likely to "power through" illness, [and more likely to] stay home, rest and recover more quickly. Some caregivers are grumpy about this, but we have seen many appreciate more quiet time home with their very young children. (Administrator, United States)*

Staff health

> *During the pandemic, I began to have time to build myself a healthier diet, specifically eating more raw [foods] and vegetables, I began to exercise more often, at least 30 minutes a day, and I also started making time to read books. Those are the activities I still want to keep because I feel so much better in my body and mind. (Educator, Vietnam)*

> *We are now more used to staying home when we feel sick and not coming out of duty when we feel bad. (Educator, Germany)*

> *I have been able to take better care of myself due to the fact that I am home much more than I was during the pandemic. I eat better because*

I cook all our meals at home. I take time to care for my body much more as I am not on the road as much. (Teacher educator, Australia)

Time. I am no longer so tightly connected to time. Time no longer has a tight grip on me. I am much more relaxed and fluid. (Assistant, United States)

I have a Waldorf home family childcare, and I reduced one hour the daily program, do parent meetings by Zoom, reduced my attendance in conference. Because I recognized that my selfcare is more important that improve the quality of day with children [sic]. (Educator, United States)

Creating a better work life balance for myself. (Educator, Canada)

Improved training and education

In the responses received, small numbers of people specifically mentioned training and being better equipped with technical skills. There were comments that "*online skills gained during Covid have given new possibilities*" (teacher educator, United Kingdom), and becoming "*much better at making online videos with assignments/stories/songs for children*" (educator, Netherlands). Educators appeared to have adapted to and adopted online communication with ease. Some participants mentioned the positive changes within the area of parent involvement which have been made possible by increased understanding of and facility with digital communications platforms, while others look forward to contact being only face to face again.

[What changes do I want to keep?] Increased online training. (Educator, Germany)

As someone who organises and contributes to adult education, both initial early childhood training and CPD, the online skills gained during Covid have given new possibilities and we have kept some sessions (not very many) online and kept our online weekly study group. (Teacher educator, United Kingdom)

The knowledge of online Waldorf resources. (Educator, United States)

The online study, I discovered that it is possible to study and do several things even if it is not possible to be presidential [sic. Present is possibly meant]. (Educator, United States)

During the pandemic, we tried running classes for students and open lectures for everyone online. We saw the impracticality of providing vocational training online. This was also confirmed by students who have been studying with us for several years. They asked us to teach the same subjects face-to-face. Which we did. Public lectures were in demand by the students. We plan to hold online lectures 2-3 times during the year. This allows us to reach a larger number of listeners and awaken interest in pedagogy. (Teacher educator, Russia)

Diversity

In May 2020, towards the start of the pandemic, Black American George Floyd was murdered by a Minneapolis police officer who suspected that he had used a forged $20 note. The protests which followed his killing led to a worldwide protest movement under the banner of Black Lives Matter. This highlighted the discrimination people of colour face at the hands of the police. Also in May 2020, it was already being acknowledged that responses to the pandemic were affecting those most vulnerable in society the strongest (Schifferes, 2020). Numerous authors have observed that the pandemic has exaggerated inequalities within societies and between countries, negatively affecting those who are poor, in substandard housing, in financial stress with insecure employment, while those who are financially comfortable, owning their own home, with a secure job (which could often be done from home) had a significantly different experience (Doetter et al., 2022).

Two US-based teacher educators specifically mentioned their awareness that the pandemic affected those most vulnerable in society, which influenced their work.

As an American teacher educator, I have to include not only the challenges of the pandemic but also of what the pandemic revealed, namely the need to directly counteract the forces of racism that have infected our country since its founding. This has been revelatory! The modifications we made to our program were dramatic during the "lockdown" time in 2020 but we are now able to continue teaching our students in person. The online classes were minimal and only happened when that was the only way to continue because of public health decrees. The benefits to the students of our in-person classes became crystal clear to our faculty in comparison to online classes, particularly in preparing new teachers for their work. The other changes we made to our curriculum in response to the racism embedded in our society we will certainly keep! (Teacher educator, United States)

Since I work primarily in adult education, I am aware of the need to be sensitive and supportive to the emotional and social needs of the adult students. In the US there is a very big conflation of the effects of the pandemic and how much more sensitive everyone is, along with the long-overdue explosion of awarenesses regarding Diversity, Equity, Inclusivity, and Access. People in general are quick to take offense both on their own behalf and on the behalf of others. This has to be navigated very sensitively and consciously. Everyone is "touchy" in some regard – with good reason. So the changes I am trying to make is to assume nothing about our shared attitudes and expectations and begin every session with every group as though we are creating our learning community of trust anew. (Teacher educator, United States)

Another side to this was given by an educator in the United States regarding her greatest challenge.

One of my challenges in Waldorf school is my language and race. White people think we are not able to be teachers just because we are Latinas. They want to put us always as assistants in a class. Even [when] we are prepared and have a Waldorf teacher training. (Educator, United States)

This response highlights issues which need to continue to be addressed within the Waldorf movement, not only in the United States.

A final word from an assistant from Slovenia on what she would like to keep from the pandemic period:

I will keep the hugs and the cuddles.

Q2 How have you viewed Waldorf early childhood education during these pandemic experiences?
(Strengths/things to change)

This question asked about overarching strengths and limitations of Waldorf education which had been perceived as it adapted to changes imposed during the greatly altered circumstances of pandemic restrictions. A number of overlapping themes were identified: how pedagogy was and was not affected, effects on children and staff, and effects on parents and communities including vaccine hesitancy.

How pedagogy was and was not affected

Many respondents emphasised how the pedagogy, principles and essence of Waldorf education – in terms of the child, parents, community – had influenced their own life during the pandemic period. The philosophy was discussed as a strength in terms of personal (teacher) growth and how an anthroposophical approach supported everyday functioning and activities with children: "The anthroposophical background of Waldorf education encouraged me personally to deal with the children in an easy-going (unbeschwert) way" (Educator, Germany).

Others presented Steiner's approach as being essentially flexible which meant that it could easily be adapted to emergency situations through "Having the freedom, through not having a rigid curriculum, to be able to meet the needs of the children coming towards us creatively and to truly support each child's development as an individual" (Educator, United Kingdom).

Some indicated that nothing had greatly changed:

> No matter what the social situation, we realised how much the same rhythm, repetition, example and imitation of Steiner education in preschool life provides a protective covering for the children and makes them feel safe and secure as they grow up. (Assistant, Japan)

> Otherwise, there were only minor changes in the daily routine with the children, as we live a very regulated and ritualised routine anyway. (Educator, Germany)

> The children came to the kindergarten as if nothing had ever happened - very familiar and without fear of contact. That encouraged us a lot! We were able to offer the children the security they so desperately needed. This is definitely based on the content of Waldorf education. (Administrator and educator, Germany)

or that flexibility was developed through the challenges as they arose:

> A strength was becoming more flexible and able to adapt to change more readily. I think the ability to adapt on the physical level led to a greater ability to be more flexible and open to change in terms of adapting to new methods and ideas in best practice. (Educator, Canada)

With others, it was hard to know how to teach 'Waldorf' when so much was altered.

> It's essential for the social/emotional peace. I don't feel like I was even able to scratch the surface of what the children needed in this realm because of the delays in interpersonal communication and coopera-

tion...It was definitely difficult to figure out how to teach "Waldorf" when everything was shut down. (Educator, United States)

Kindergarten education was not very good. When we could come, there were fewer of us, so the group was not the real image of the group, nor could it provide the social space for the children who came. (Educator, Hungary)

What was effective

Respondents emphasised the maintenance of rhythm and routine, the use of the outdoor environment, and a focus on emotional well-being and building resilience in activities. Through this, "*Waldorf education was able to adapt to adverse circumstances and still maintain high quality*" *(Educator, Germany)*, by "*being very flexible, not always sticking to old habits.*" *(Educator, Germany)*

The majority of educators believed Waldorf Education enabled them to manage the routine and rhythm of everyday activities during, and post-pandemic, with ease. Aspects of rhythm and routine were highlighted by educators from numerous countries.

Rhythm, routine and the outdoors

The many things that could be maintained strengthened the children and the teaching staff, such as rhythm, rituals in the daily-weekly-yearly cycle, artistic and craft activities such as watercolour painting, kneading beeswax, felting, woodwork, gardening, puppet shows, morning circles, making music, singing and much more. (Educator, Germany)

Along with the importance of maintaining rhythm for children, whether at kindergarten or at home, came the importance of the outdoors.

Our strength is in our connection to the outdoors. Movement in nature has been so healing for disregulated children. Our rhythm has also been so helpful in orientating children into and through their kindergarten days. Parents spoke about how important it was for them to set a rhythm in 'lockdown' to help smooth transitions and keep a structure to their days. Our focus on self-directed play has given children the time and the space to process their experiences. (Educator, New Zealand).

Our program became mostly an outdoor program during the pandemic for the safety/well-being of the children. Our school has been a safe haven for the children during difficult times because they have been able to remain in a daily rhythm/routine and be with their friends and enjoy the wonderful outdoors. (Administrator and educator, United States).

Well-being, soul health

As in the New Zealand extract above, educators from India and South Africa see contact with nature as essentially health giving, going out of their way to incorporate additional time in nature to counteract the restrictions present in other parts of children's lives.

My view of Waldorf early childhood education during the pandemic with all the restrictions and protocols, has been that it is for maintaining soul health in the child. It is a healing modality that enriches the child's life on every level and brings wholeness. During the pandemic I felt a need to change my approach and work far more closely with the Earth element, providing opportunities for children to experience nature, play in nature, take children out on walks to natural environments. My view is that this is essential to their healing from the effects of the pandemic. (Educator, South Africa)

The absence of contact with the outdoors during lockdown was especially difficult for children with special needs.

It was a great challenge to work with autistic or special needs children, while the regular kids went back to hometowns. The special needs children were finding it difficult to cope inside the four walls of a house. (Educator, India)

The effects on children and staff

There was emphasis on educators' ability (or lack of ability) to connect or bond with children when wearing a mask or while trying to maintain distance, specifically in terms of security, care, empathy, support and presence. At the same time, respondents acknowledged ways in which their own well-being had been affected and that they were themselves in need of soul care.

Masks, contact

Education without seeing the adult's facial expression is very complicated for 2–6-year-olds. Facial expressions play a fundamental role in both academic and social learning. Not being able to take a crying child in one's arms to console him or her is horrible for both the child and the adult. It is also an uncomfortable position for the peers because the child cries longer and the example given by the adult is that the child has to calm down by himself. When you are three years old, it is a complicated thing and so sad! (Educator, France)

Contact bans/restrictions/controls/disinfectants/face masks and Waldorf education are mutually exclusive. (Educator, Germany)

With young children, personal contact is the key, you can't always tell stories on the computer instead, you can't play circle games alone, you can't connect communally during play. These, intimacy, physical contact are the strengths, you can't change that. (Educator, Hungary)

Educators

I don't feel like I was even able to scratch the surface of what the children needed … because of the delays in interpersonal communication and cooperation... It was definitely difficult to figure out how to teach "Waldorf" when everything was shut down. (Educator, United States)

Somewhat rebellious, difficult to adjust to and implement new things. (Administrator and educator, Germany)

Effects on parents and communities

A number of responses highlighted the two-sided nature of lockdown experiences. What some experienced as calm moments of family time together, allowing for high-quality interaction—which was widely reported early on in the pandemic (Boland & Mortlock, 2020)—others experienced as high-stress.

Families were together, they ate dinner together, they didn't leave home, they looked after each other. Strange as it may seem, it had a very good effect on the kindergarten children! (Educator, Hungary)

During the isolation period, some families experienced the stress of educating two or more of their own children which meant those with large families didn't always have the time to follow experiences suggested by teachers as the focus was needed to support their older children with their home packages. (Educator, Australia)

There was a lot of stress and anxiety in the families, and this affected the children. (Educator, Hungary)

There has needed to be an intervention to support teachers with counselling and PD to help deal with anxiety and overwhelm. Large-scale school community events have now begun again but the resilience of staff is being worn down and teachers are less able to take on tasks willingly. Negative feedback is taken to heart and comes across as harsh and finger pointing. Keeping the classes calm and slow with a strong rhythm has been more important than ever, and yet also more challenging. The children have returned with the influence of media very obvious in the play and interactions. Play and games often comes from computer games and images and social interaction suffers when the other children are unaware of the game rules or expectations. Free play needs more nurturing now. The children often seem to need to be entertained and get bored a lot more. Children seem more needy of attention and there is a need to teach sharing and kindness. There is a feeling of anger rising easily when things don't go the way that most children want. (Administrator, Australia)

Pedagogy defends itself if it is only possible to work in the real world, if kindergartens are closed then the difficulty is in "remote teaching". In this case, in my opinion, the most important thing is to contact the parents and give them tips and materials so that they can use this as an aid, an inspiration in caring for their children. (Educator, Poland)

Parents were closer to the content and methods of Waldorf pedagogy because of the pandemic. (Educator, Romania)

Vaccine hesitancy

Vaccine hesitancy in Waldorf communities was well documented before the Covid-19 pandemic occurred. For instance, in Sweden, Byström and others (2014) note that, while a wide range of opinions on vaccination is held by Waldorf parents, "Anthroposophic communities in Europe are one of several groups with relatively low vaccination coverage." Further, these communities are able to be divided into four main groupings: "*the conformers*, the *pragmatists* and the *attentive delayers*" who vaccinate their children, and the "*promoters of natural immunity*" (p. 6754, italics original) who do not. Sobo (2015, 2016) points out that identification with anthroposophy is not key to vaccine refusal, but rather that there is a "socially cultivated nature of vaccine refusal in Waldorf school settings" (2015, p. 381) guided by "school community norms." Into this might now be added the influence of social media.
Kaastan (2021) notes that

> Vaccine hesitant parents in the United States, like the United King-dom, are typically highly educated and heavily invested in their

children's health, often researching vaccinations thoroughly and resorting to refusal as a strategy to care for and to protect their children (Kaufman 2010; Leach and Fairhead 2007; Poltorak et al. 2005; Reich 2014; Sobo 2015). The social processes through which parents make vaccine decisions then conflict with public health representations of non-vaccination as a social risk. (p. 412)

In Dornach, the Medical Section at the Goetheanum put out a statement before the pandemic began, stating that "Anthroposophic Medicine is not anti-vaccine and does not support anti-vaccine movements" (2019, April 15). This was supplemented during the pandemic by a further statement from the International Federation of Anthroposophic Medical Associations (IVAA) and the Medical Section of the Goetheanum.

Voluntary vaccination

We see voluntary vaccination as a fundamental right of democratic societies and a prerequisite for a high level of acceptance among the population, not least given the remaining questions concerning efficacy and safety. A free vaccination decision requires detailed information and the opportunity to ask questions, preferably in a trusting patient-physician relationship but even during mass vaccination. In addition policy makers should prevent scenarios of indirect vaccination obligations, such as by employers, insurers or transport companies. (2021)

In some countries during the Covid-pandemic, most notably Germany, there was extensive negative publicity (Escritt, 2021) around the vaccination stance of some associated with the anthroposophical movement (not necessarily from Waldorf communities) which is seen as having a negative impact on the reputation of Waldorf education overall (Selg, 2021). While some involved in Waldorf education also took part in the extended protests against vaccine mandates in New Zealand for example (New Zealand Herald, 2022), there was no discernible negative coverage involving anthroposophy or Waldorf education.

Comments made around vaccines and vaccination within the second questionnaire include:

I experienced that Waldorf education in particular was viewed very critically by the public and there was also hostility. For example, things like "mask refusal", "Corona deniers" and "vaccination opponents" were topics. I found it very helpful that the [German] Association of Waldorf Kindergartens repeatedly took a stand on these issues and that they were conveyed to the outside world. In our institution, as the director, I placed a lot of emphasis on the strict implementation of all the prescribed measures - this was not always easy and there were many conflicts within the teaching staff and the parents. Nevertheless, we have grown very much as a community and have always been able to discuss things constructively. Our institution got through the pandemic without any group closures or notable absences – we showed a lot of consideration for the concerns and needs of the parents and offered emergency groups throughout. Waldorf education should have distanced itself even more from the negative accusations – that would certainly have been helpful for the individual institutions. (Educator, Germany)

There was a great divide between vaccination opponents and vaccination supporters. This has affected the whole of life. Friendships broke up. Parents even left the kindergarten. I experienced this massive antagonism mainly in the Waldorf sector. In other areas of society there was not as much attention paid to pro or contra vaccination as in Waldorf kindergartens. Also, being in the pandemic, which was otherwise so positive, limited us, because, at first, we didn't know any ways to work online. We had to learn that first. (Educator, Germany)

It was very hard. Each family's reactions weren't the same. Some of them were very scared, some of them just believed in vaccine. …If [the educator] thinks that the children are sick, they are sent home. We tried to open the windows often. (Educator, Romania)

The strength [of Waldorf education] is that, no matter what happens, we can be sure of what is important for the development of children and adults. I felt how important it is to have a simple and rhythmic life. What needs to change: Many people involved in Steiner education have a negative view of vaccination, but I think that there is an option to receive vaccination knowing the disadvantages when looking at it from the perspective of being born in the Corona era and living together while also being connected to society. It is also necessary to respond flexibly to social trends without being overly biased. (Educator, Japan)

I'm curious about all the talk of childhood illness and the importance of building an immune system and how readily so many in the greater Waldorf community were proponents of masking and vaccines. (Educator, United States)

We did not see any signs of anxiety among the children or hear any concerns from their parents. However, opinions were divided on vaccination, and the anthroposophical doctor shared his opinion with all staff and parents. I have my own values and beliefs, but sometimes I have to *make decisions in the circumstances of the moment. I found it important to think and respond flexibly while learning more. (Educator, Japan)*

We are so flexible and resilient! I am so proud of how we were able to make our program into a fully outdoor program (except for nap) to avoid forcing the young ones to wear masks. I am a little discouraged at the governance of our school that put great amounts of pressure on the students and employees to get the Covid vaccinations. I realize that was also state driven, living in California, but there was quite a bit of pressure. (Educator, United States)

Although most kindergartens are back to some kind of normal, it is likely that collegial and community rifts caused by the divisive nature of governmental vaccination policies are not yet healed and could break open again if a similar situation arises. Similarly, the negative publicity which anthroposophy and Waldorf education received in mainstream media in some countries (not necessarily tied to kindergartens) will need to be countered.

There was a repeated belief stated that the Waldorf principles and 'usual' routine ensured that students had better immunity and were healthier compared to other children:

I reaffirmed that the practice of Steiner early childhood education makes children healthy, and this has given me confidence in my own practice. (Educator, Japan)

Children do not wear masks, but few are infected. I believe this is the result of building up their immunity through a life of Steiner early childhood education. (Administrator, Japan)

No studies have been made to support such a claim. A similar claim about increased immunity was made about working with anthroposophy.

I think we should focus on working with parents and strengthening our immunity through regular classes in anthroposophy. (Educator, Russia)

Another comment about the importance of anthroposophy included:

...anthroposophy is even more necessary at this moment. Without anthroposophical understanding and practice it would be much more unconscious and unhealthy in this period in which I live. I see an adaptation of the language as necessary. Anthroposophy is profound: it needs to be. But the language used with families needs to be simpler. We need, as teachers, to develop empathy with the challenges of each family that arrives. What needs to change is a certain distancing of

teachers or a lack of acceptance of the real situation in each home. We need to deal with people in a real way, idealizing them takes us away from fruitful pedagogical work. (Educator, Brazil)

Q3 What is the most important thing you have learned from the pandemic experience?

Responses to this question are perhaps the most insightful and forwards looking. So many pandemic experiences have been challenging and disruptive; what has been learned for the future is less frequently the focus of attention. Some respondents highlighted an increased awareness of the importance of looking after one's own well-being, remaining calm, being adaptable and open to change, and cultivating inner resilience. Others focused on relationships and community, strengthening connections after what has been for many a divisive period.

Self-care and personal growth

A significant number of respondents mentioned the importance to them of being connected to the principles of Waldorf education and anthroposophy and of the support gained by inner work. This could be through "*maintaining trust in spiritual guidance and accompaniment, and strengthening myself through prayer*" (Educator, Germany) or in that "*I can draw meaning and strength from anthroposophy and Steiner education as if from a spring of life … [in order] to live more consciously in connection with the spiritual helpers, the angelic world, and to appreciate the beauty, truth and goodness in everything small. Cultivate gratitude*" (Educator, Switzerland).

For some, a key learning in this disruptive period was the value of prioritising their own mental health and well-being and spending more time with their own families; details were shared of personal struggles, breakthroughs and insights, learning to "*live healthily, love yourself, your family and society, and [spend] more time with family*" (Educator, Vietnam). The role of being a participatory and responsible individual within the community was also mentioned, including the importance to individual well-being of being linked to the community: "*I learned how much it means to be part of a collective, how much support and strength it gives you to be part of a collective of people, that you are not alone, and how much physical encounters between people, face-to-face conversations, … gestures, [and] warmth of soul matter*" (Teacher educator, Romania).

The most prominent learning across responses was the ability to be calm, resilient and adaptable if the need arose. Such an attitudinal shift included the importance of learning to "*go with the flow*", "*improvise*", "*find* a rhythm", "learn to switch quickly", "to be simple", with "flexibility and resourcefulness". There was also emphasis placed on the value of "breaking free" from accustomed and familiar ways of teaching and being open to new ways of working.

Inner well-being

I can draw meaning and strength from anthroposophy and Steiner education as if from a spring of life. I can develop my own courage and strength. I have learned that together with colleagues and parents we can live more positively. And that crises are connected to a task that can be solved together. (Educator, Switzerland)

[What I have learned is] To ask questions, to do research and to trust what feels best. To remember how important the four lower senses[3] are in early childhood and how we meet the children. How very important touch is! (Educator, United States)

A counter picture was also given to this.

Experiencing Waldorf educators who have lost their basic trust in the spiritual world (Teacher educator, Canada)

It would be worthwhile investigating if this loss of trust is experienced widely and what stands behind it, or if it is an isolated instance.

Attitude

This experience has reinforced the essential element of human connection. It is the main work of our time to meet the other with an open and accepting heart, with reverence and respect, and with the true intention of understanding them on a deep level. (Educator, United States)

Don't forget to take care of yourself and your colleagues. (Educator, United States)

Being patient with myself. (Educator, India)

To be flexible and follow the children's lead. Relationships really are central to Waldorf education and the more we can find that human essence in our teaching, the better. (Educator, United States)

---

3 The sense of touch, sense of life, sense of movement and sense of balance. For further details on the senses, see Soesman, 1990.

Communication and relationship

The importance of relationships came out further in comments about communication and interaction with parents and community, and how these had been affected during the pandemic. Educators indicated some good practices which had proved successful and which they intended keeping in the future, such as *"Giving parents and colleagues as much information as possible, including the information that I don't know the answer to a question. Try to communicate as clearly as possible"* (Administrator and educator, Czechia). Furthermore, the centrality of communication for healthy relationships was expressed in different ways. *"Communication is everything. I rang every family every week. I actually got to know the families more intimately than in a usual school year. I offered support and encouraged local meet-ups"* (Educator, Switzerland). The realisation of the need to communicate more effectively overlapped with a need for a shift in attitude in some instances: [I've learned] *"That it is necessary to be open to different points of view and always try to find a way that is good for [everyone]"* (Educator, Slovenia). In some cases, educators expressed heightened gratitude for the possibility of interacting face to face again: *"I approach my collegial relationships with more compassion and humour than before. It feels like living through the pandemic has really crystalized my love for this important work and its innate therapeutic and healing qualities"* (Educator, United States).

A few educators mentioned the ability to use online resources with increased ease and how this has contributed to their learning: *"We also learned about the possibility of sharing resources on-line and about all the wonderful schools out there in the world to whom we now feel more of a connection having met via Zoom"* (Educator, Canada) and *"I think that what this change of life has left us with is the realisation that we can support each other no matter where [we] are or what [we] want to share by Zooming around the world"* (Assistant, Mexico).

Interaction and involvement of and with parents and community

Human warmth is a priority, to be maintained absolutely, even if one is limited in touch etc. Relationship with children and parents is paramount. (Educator, Switzerland)

This experience has reinforced the essential element of human connection. It is the main work of our time to meet the other with an open and [accepting] heart, with reverence and respect, and with the true intention of understanding them on a deep level. (Educator, United States)

> *Relationships with children, families and between families are most important in weathering and learning from difficult times. (Educator, United States)*

Some mentioned that what they had learned was around the human failings.

> *The parental community is very important but is becoming weaker and weaker. Everyone focuses on their own child...Much insecurity among adults. (Educator, Switzerland)*

> *Fear spreads quickly. (Administrator and educator, Australia)*

But that it is necessary and possible to work through these.

> *The world is connected. It is also important to think about how to deal with people who think differently. (Educator, Japan)*

> *I learned that the small child, despite the rules and regulation, loved coming to school. That children love to learn regardless of the circumstance. (Educator, South Africa)*

> *It is much more important to ensure that childcare is soothing in the midst of a pandemic, that a calm and serene environment and loving care are provided. (Administrator, Japan).*

Q4 What is the single greatest challenge you face?

Regarding the challenges faced by those in Waldorf early childhood settings, the attitude and role of parents was frequently highlighted, in terms of the behaviours which children had grown used to during lockdown, habits they had adopted, parents' indifference to the Waldorf approach, and children being withdrawn, for whatever reason, from kindergartens. Beyond the challenges of lockdown and mask wearing, emphasis was placed on the difficulty of adapting the learning environment to an altered mindset and lifestyle of children, while ensuring that their developmental needs were met. There was also repeated mention of ideological differences and tensions caused when trying to uphold the Waldorf approach while, at the same time, complying with government mandates.

Although not everyone found that new challenges had arisen, "*[the challenges] have not changed from the time before Corona*" (Educator, Netherlands), overall, four themes emerged: people and community, creating a safe and healthy learning environment, time pressures and processes, and laws and regulations.

People and community

One of the main challenges which respondents highlighted was a noticeable change in parental attitudes, involvement and support compared to before the pandemic. This took the form of reduced participation,

> *Bringing communities back together. Volunteering is decreasing. As a result, the quality within Waldorf institutions is suffering. (Administrator and educator, Germany)*

> *Decreasing parental interest and involvement in children's education (Educator, Romania)*

as well as an apparent lack of confidence in or support for educators.

> *Regain the confidence of parents. (Educator, Switzerland)*

> *Parents lack of care and thought for our staff... This has put us into chaos and created a lot of hurt... We recently had a meeting where the staff were feeling very despondent and not feeling appreciated by our community. Listening to them I suggested that, once more, if we wanted to turn this around it was going to have to come from us, even though we are feeling exhausted. (Administrator and educator, New Zealand)*

Dealing with difference

As indicated on page 77, the subject of vaccination within anthroposophical and Waldorf circles had been the topic of study before the Covid pandemic began (e.g. Sobo, 2015), highlighting the different opinions held. Government-imposed restrictions and mandates increased the range and strength of these differences, with viewpoints becoming increasingly polarised. This had a strong effect on kindergartens, their staff and communities (see page 77). Though the large majority of mandates now have been withdrawn, the after-effects of the polarisation are still felt.

For some, the lasting effects of this polarisation were the greatest challenges they are currently facing.

> *Dealing with the different views within anthroposophy and the free school [Waldorf school] on measures and vaccinations. That's where real misunderstanding and friction arose. I was really bothered by dogmatic images from anthroposophy, the condemnation if you do get tested and vaccinated, and want to adhere to government policies. I found that the most difficult. (Educator, Netherlands)*

[Dealing with] dogmatic Waldorf teachers, administrators and Waldorf Schools!!! (Administrator, United States)

The divisiveness in the community. (Educator, New Zealand)

Objections from those that disagree with how we handle things. (Educator, United States)

Remarks about the importance of tolerance, calm, acceptance, working on yourself, not being judgmental (previous question) are obviously key learnings here. "*Putting one's own attitude aside and reacting professionally in difficult situations with difficult measures, such as wearing a mask while teaching, etc.*" (Educator, Switzerland) becomes an important attribute.

Financial stresses

The Covid-19 pandemic had almost immediate effects on the lives and livelihoods of people all over the globe. As lockdowns were put into effect, millions of people lost their jobs and, with it, financial security. Others had significant wage reductions. Many countries implemented financial support packages which offset these measures to some degree. Despite this financial support, the day-to-day finances of many parents suffered and the rolls of some kindergartens fell (see the graph on page 51) which impacted the financial health and sometimes viability of centres (Noble, 2020). Following the lifting of lockdowns, significant numbers of people are still suffering from financial stress, in part due to lasting consequences of the pandemic, the war in Ukraine and abrupt rises in the cost of living (Timmins & Thomas, 2022). This continues to impact the rolls of kindergartens negatively and remains a challenge for educators in many countries, especially those which do not receive state support.

There was a reduction in the number of children enrolled this year, due to the requirement of proof of vaccination, for the collective good, which consequently generated financial challenges, together with a reduction of voluntary contributions of families, also due to reductions in family income. (Administrator and educator, Brazil).

There have been financial implications for our school related to the pandemic, and we have also experienced difficulty maintaining adequate staffing. (Educator, Canada).

[Our challenge is] making sure classes get fuller again. Many people have moved out of town for more space, classes are running empty. (Educator, Netherlands)

For Waldorf School[s] to survive in this country is hard. I see many people want this education, but they can't afford it on top of increasing living costs. (Educator, United States)

This situation also impacts teacher education courses.

As a result of restrictions and job losses, people have less opportunity to come to study. The number of students has more than halved during this time. Hence the seminar has a financial problem. (Teacher educator, Russia)

For our TT [teacher training] program, time will tell. Our enrollment is quite low, and we can bridge this year but it's not sustainable long-term. (Teacher educator, United States)

Additionally, there are signs that, at least in some countries, this is not going to get better in the short term.

The cost-of-living crisis is going to mean that families cannot afford the fees in our schools and numbers will probably drop. At the same time, we already have a recruitment crisis partly because the salaries are so low that EC teachers cannot afford to live on them. This is going to become more acute in the next two years and we may see Kindergartens close due to lack of staff. (Teacher educator, United Kingdom).

Safe/healthy environment

A task of any kindergarten is to ensure that the environment it provides makes educators, parents and children feel relaxed and secure. Several educators cited that the single biggest challenge is *"to find a good approach to the pandemic and general health that makes each staff member, parents and children feel comfortable and safe"* (educator, Germany). There was emphasis on the difficulty in drawing children back into the physical spaces to learn and engage, while increased exposure to digital technologies at home during the pandemic, both for learning and used as a distraction or entertainment, has had a negative influence on the children generally: *"How can I ensure that young children play with real things as much as possible and not be presented with all kinds of videos and games?"* (Educator, Netherlands).

Another challenge is a discernible weakening of children's ability (and wish) to play and engage with other children. *"The biggest challenge I am finding is that children are asking for too much exclusivity, they always need an adult with them, watching what they do, playing together. I believe that the pandemic has brought this about because of the social isolation and the little ones often prefer the company of an adult rather than another child"*

(Educator, Brazil). This also included the question of how to respond with activities to such behavioural changes – *"how we will resume our activities after the pandemic has settled down?" (Educator, Japan).*

Need for socialisation

Waldorf educators around the world reported that children find it harder to play with others, especially those who do not have siblings (Hinsliff, 2022) and want more individual attention from the adults in the room. (Solo parents faced additional challenges during lockdowns as well.) Peer-mediated emotional regulation has not been able to take place to the same degree as pre-pandemic and children show reduced tolerance to the views of others or willingness to accept not 'getting their own way'. Additionally, children from disadvantaged and marginalised backgrounds are more likely to have a particularly challenging time (Fegert et al., 2020).

> *Now that we are back in school and have contact with children who experienced the pandemic in a different way, the challenge is to offer them the tools so that they can heal what the confinement has caused them, such as the lack of socialisation, working with language, tolerance to frustration, etc. (Kindergarten assistant, Mexico)*

> *The biggest challenge I am finding is that children are asking for too much exclusivity, they always need an adult with them, watching what they do, playing together. I believe that the pandemic has brought this about because of the social isolation and the little ones often prefer the company of an adult rather than another child. (Educator, Brazil)*

> *Some children no longer play freely with others; they always need the presence and attention of an adult. (Teacher educator, Romania)*

> *I work with a large group of children who have come out of two years of social isolation. This has affected their social, emotional and physical development in significant ways. In particular they have found it very difficult to adapt to a large social group. They have a higher sense of entitlement and lack patience and empathy towards other children. (Educator, Australia)*

> *At the moment, the after-effects of the confinement on our children, some of them were in total isolation and do not know how to relate to their peers. (Educator, Mexico)*

The effect of digital technologies

During periods of lockdowns, children were often confined to the house or apartment where they lived, in some countries this meant not being allowed outside (in the case of Spain, children could not go outside for six weeks, see World Economic Forum, 2020). Some in apartments did not have ready access to gardens or other open spaces during this time. Parents worldwide turned increasingly to digital media to fill the gap left by previous human interaction and contact, partly as baby-sitting or entertainment, partly as educational tool (Bergmann et al., 2022). This was also the case in Waldorf circles, though perhaps less widespread than elsewhere.

The absence of digital technologies is a defining feature of Steiner kindergartens (Nicol & Taplin, 2017); instead, simple technologies are used which "reveal their working principles on the outside and in use" (p. 155). Numerous respondents noted that rebalancing the digital and 'real' is currently their main challenge, post-pandemic.

> *The world is becoming increasingly digital. How can I ensure that young children play with real things as much as possible and not be presented with all kinds of videos and games? (Educator, Netherlands)*

> *… children going back to school show signs of the influence of electronic devices. (Educator, Vietnam)*

> *To cultivate cooperation with the parents in such a way that together we can transform the strong negative influence of the digital screen world and the increasing dependence on it into a consciously different way of thinking and acting, so that the children can grow up healthily and their incarnation is made possible undisturbed. (Educator, Germany)*

> *[Set] boundaries for digital use. (Educator, Japan)*

Fear and anxiety

One of the consequences of the Covid pandemic which has been well documented is the increase in anxiety across populations, which is in turn picked up by young children (Radanović et al., 2021; Sancho et al., 2021; Viola & Nunes) who themselves become fearful. Mitigating the anxieties and fears which children (and others) carry was found in educators' responses from a wide range of countries.

> *New habits take a long time to introduce. Habits that came from the fear-based interpretation of the illness caused by the Covid virus are seen as good. However, the underlying fear has brought an element*

into the habit that is not built on respect. "Wash your hands otherwise I might become sick!" instead of "Wash your hands sparkling and clean for our next task to become sparkling too." The unspoken thread penetrated deeply! "Keep distance, you are too close!" It is a daily task to bring trust as a mood to the children. (Educator, South Africa)

Developmental delays, emotional regulation difficulties, anxiety and social difficulties. Almost all the children in the group face one difficulty or another from the above list. (Educator, Israel)

The biggest challenge for me is the parents with their fears that they pass on to their children. (Educator, Netherlands)

Understanding and transforming/resolving the increased insecurity, anxiety, reticence and anger/aggression of the children/others. (Educator, Germany)

Now I'm just working hard to restore natural behaviour and create a fear-free environment for children and adults. (Educator, Denmark)

That we can let the children in in all warmth without having to be fearful of each other. (Educator, Norway)

We take care to talk to the children and to their parents and guardians in a way that they do not feel anxious, so that they can live in the school with peace of mind and a cheerful face. (Educator, Japan)

To bring the joy of life and confidence to children and parents again and again. (Educator, Germany)

Masks

Requirements to teach while wearing a mask and ensure that young children wear masks in the kindergarten proved to be an emotive issue in many countries, with conflicting opinions also voiced by professionals (for example Esposito & Principi, 2020; Huppertz et al., 2021; Stajduhar et al., 2022). In 2022, staff at the University of Witten/Herdecke in Germany (Schwarz et al., 2021) published the initial results of a registry set up for parents to record the effects of children wearing masks – likely containing entries by many Waldorf parents – the first self-reporting register for such a purpose. While multiple negative effects were reported, including "irritability (60%), headache (53%), difficulty concentrating (50%), less happiness (49%), reluctance to go to school/kindergarten (44%), malaise (42%) impaired learning (38%) and drowsiness or fatigue (37%)", the article states that "Due to multiple limitations[4], this study cannot demon-

---

4 Including being "distributed preferentially in social media fora that, according to the authors, 'criticize the government's corona protection measures in principle'" and containing "sampling bias, reporting bias, and confounding bias as well as lack of a control group."

strate a causal relationship between mask wearing and the reported adverse effects in children" (p. 355).

Under challenges faced, respondents mentioned masks and mask mandates, in particular, the lack of face-to-face contact and its possible lasting effects (see Stajduhar et al., 2022), and the divisiveness which came into many kindergarten communities through opposing viewpoints.

When our school got sucked into the division of masks/not-masks, vaccines/not-vaccines, this almost divided our community, but since we held each other in love, now we are stronger, though some have left to join other schools and more have joined ours. (Educator, Canada)

We have also had to learn to deal with differences in views which could even be extreme (masking, vaccines...). (Educator, Canada)

Fortunately, our parents were not too particular about the mask recommendation. One family even announced that if we all wore masks, they would keep their child at home. (Administrator, Finland)

[My biggest challenge is] some people thinking Covid is a joke and not wanting to wear a mask. (Educator, New Zealand)

A Swiss educator explained the predicament this created, and the importance of

Putting one's own attitude aside and reacting professionally in difficult situations, with difficult measures such as wearing the mask while teaching, etc. (Educator, Switzerland)

The effects or possible effects on children were stressed by others.

Compulsory vaccination, compulsory masks, keeping a distance, exaggerated hygiene requirements are contrary to the basic human needs for closeness, touch, basic trust. This is what I struggle with the most. (Educator, Germany)

We saw that with small children masks were a problem because they could not see our faces and could not hear us properly. (Administrator, Finland)

The children spend the daytime without masks, but the caregivers wear masks and are constantly concerned about how this affects the physical and mental development required in early childhood, such as not being able to see the caregivers' facial expressions. For individuals, the biggest challenges are overcoming the suffocation of masked childcare (especially during morning circle and story time) in the summer heat. (Educator, Japan)

Wearing a mask is troublesome, I'm unable to speak softly, children can't hear clearly, and it is easier [for them] to stay in their own world. They are more reluctant to participate in common activities. (Educator, Taiwan)

Although the situation has eased, we are required to hold parents' [meetings] online...this development is a pity as it prevents intensive cooperation...parents' meetings have to be conducted with a mask. A lot of things can't be conveyed that way, because it needs facial expression! (Educator, Brazil)

Time and processes

This section includes the challenges of new procedures, shifts in approach and the pressure to manage these changes. There were mentions of the stresses and pressure caused by following changing rules, managing work-life balance, and implementing the pedagogy to the best of the staff's abilities.

Dealing with ever-changing requirements and demands, coming from outside government and society, dealing with stressed people and preventing myself from becoming overloaded and stressed too. (Administrator and educator, New Zealand).

References to challenges with being able to implement the Waldorf approach within the limitations of not only Covid regulations:

How to deliver the wonderful richness of Steiner early years education within the rigid and horrid demands from the framework that is the EYFS in England. (Educator, United Kingdom).

Time poverty and the results of not having enough time were mentioned as a challenge for the educators:

The biggest challenge is not to overextend ourselves even more. This is difficult because now that the situation has eased, there should be more time for self-care and follow-up or processing what has happened. But somehow there isn't. Sometimes I feel so out of sorts that I don't feel like a human being anymore - many people feel that way. (Administrator and educator, Germany)

Finding the time. As life has opened up again, it has become busy, if not busier. (Educator, United Kingdom)

To bring the whole rhythm into place post-pandemic took almost three times the effort, time and skill. How to ease such a task is the biggest challenge. (Educator, India).

Others concentrated more on what is to come next.

> *I wasted a lot of time thinking about how my classroom will never be the same instead of brainstorming new ideas on how to bring the community and warmth into the classroom in a new safe way. (Educator, United States)*

> *Fighting back for the rights of pre-schoolers in the larger community of the school. Not just going back to pre-pandemic times but looking critically and communicating strongly enough to colleagues. (Educator, Belgium)*

> *I think it is also important to try to learn lessons from what has happened. Sometimes it seems that we have stepped right back into the rat race, whereas we actually cherished the imposed slowdown during the pandemic so much. (Educator, Belgium)*

Laws and regulations

Throughout the Covid-19 pandemic, restrictions and increased regulations were imposed by governments and health departments on all sectors of society, including early childhood education. There was an emphasis on the use of social distancing, enhanced hygiene, masks and vaccines. These regulations differed from country to country, state to state and from month to month. In many cases, they put stresses on parents, educators and administrators alike, which came on top of other stresses caused by the pandemic. Additionally, they served to exacerbate longer-held grievances and dissatisfactions (McClure, 2022). An increase in anxiety and fear was widespread in children, parents (Tatsiopoulou et al., 2022) and educators (Sparks, 2022). Accustomed practices in kindergartens were not possible. At one stage, singing was prohibited in Australian schools and kindergartens in New South Wales (NSW Government, 2020), something which hit Steiner institutions hard (Boland, 2020a).

The reception of these restrictions and regulations varied greatly. As previously stated, communities became divided, friendships were broken, children were withdrawn from kindergartens, and non-vaccinated educators had to leave or were made redundant. Health requirements and sound pedagogy frequently came into conflict, a tension which educators and administrators had to live within every day (in addition to the stresses of their own personal lives). Issues of bio-politics (Foucault et al., 2008) became everday topics of discussion and debate within Steiner settings as elsewhere. Questions of ethics, the balance between private and public, between individual freedom and public good, between positive freedoms and negative freedoms (Redaelli, 2020), and the ethics of being 'tracked' by Covid apps (Farina & Lavazza, 2021) all became hotly contested topics of conversation and, sometimes, protest (Gillespie & Breen, 2021; James et al., 2022).

These responses were given under 'greatest challenge'.

The bureaucratic apparatus as opposed to pedagogy consumes too much time and energy. (Educator, Germany)

Organising all the changes that were coming from the government that could every day be different - and that created lots of stress for all of the staff - every day. Not knowing what to expect! So, to give the children good care, we were exhausted after five hours every day without having possibilities to take a break. (Administrator and educator, Norway).

The guidelines and laws imposed by the state, which in no way represent a responsible approach to basic human needs. (Educator, Germany).

External pressures. That certain constraints become the norm to which we should adapt. (Educator, Czechia)

Around the world, there have been protests by those who believe that their governments have overstepped their role and become autocratic. In other countries, there have been protests about governments approaching the pandemic too laxly, leaving what is a societal health emergency to the individual. The tensions between these have led some voicing protest at the feeling of always being told what to do.

I am annoyed by any AUTOCRATIC / HIERARCHICAL approach. It doesn't matter if by the government, colleagues, parents... Even the norms are not "friendly" to our work... (Educator, Slovenia)

Getting back into the boat together and throwing off dead weight. (Administrator and educator, Germany)

Staffing

One of the strongest impacts of these regulations was the imposition of vaccination mandates on various professions, including education (all sectors). Refusal to be vaccinated meant that people had to leave their jobs or they were made redundant. These forced redundancies affected some countries more than others, and has exacerbated reported staff shortages, as well as resulting in the loss of experienced colleagues.

Relief staffing. The continuing grief of parents who lost two of their teachers through the vaccine mandates. (Educator, New Zealand)

The divide created in our school community – pro-mask/vax versus anti-mask/vax...We lost more than 50% of our enrollment and many of our teachers left. (Educator, United States)

My biggest challenge is finding good staff. (Educator, Germany)

These were some of themes which emerged from the concerns raised by respondents to the survey. It is not possible to detail them all. What appears strongly is that responses are broadly similar no matter which continent they come from. It is apparent that experiences of Steiner kindergarten staff of the Covid-19 pandemic are to a substantial degree consistent across countries and across cultures.

Conclusion

The Covid-19 pandemic has been a unique and incisive event in the personal and professional lives of everyone reading this report. We have all been affected by the policies enacted by our governments over the past three years. While these policies may have been appropriate to contain the outbreak, reduce mortality and minimise pressure on national health systems, they came at a cost. The pandemic raised exceptional, unanticipated challenges for which kindergartens and their staff were unprepared. On top of dealing with the consequences of the pandemic on a personal level, which possibly included the loss of close family members and friends, ill health, financial insecurity, and chronic uncertainty and stress, those working in Steiner early childhood education had the added responsibility of caring for young children and their families.

This report has attempted to bring out pertinent themes from the data given by respondents to the surveys. The data produced is rich and gives a broad overview of experiences of those working in Steiner early childhood education at this time. It is a snapshot of opinion and experience in September 2022. Responses could well be different if the same questions were asked now. This breadth covers those working in Steiner early childhood education around and across the world. It offers a rare opportunity to hear the voices and experiences of those working in similar occupations but in different geographies and circumstances.

Drawing conclusions from data of this richness is a challenge; there is so much to talk about. It is beyond the scope of this report to travel down the many avenues of further inquiry indicated in the data or drill down into individual national responses. Some of these will be explored in additional publications. However, at the risk of omitting important threads, I am going to highlight two broad themes which emerge from the study. The first is well-being, the second change and responsivity.

Well-being

The first section of the first questionnaire asked eight questions about well-being. All were reported to be less positive than before the pandemic. This is likely not a surprise given all that has happened since the start of 2020. However, within this, it is comment worthy how often well-being was referred to in different ways in the replies given to Questionnaire 2. Steiner's 'pedagogical law' (1924/1998)[5] makes it clear that children's well-being is strongly affected by the well-being of those adults around them. Healthy and well-regulated educators help create healthy and well-regulated children. The greatest number of responses to the question, *what is the most important thing you have learned from the pandemic experience?* (Q3) involved ways found to enhance well-being in some way, including renewed understanding of and respect for the basic measure of not trying to go into work when unwell, caring for oneself as well as for others, the importance of nourishing one's inner life and of being part of a community.

Well-being also applies to communities around Steiner kindergartens. A consistent theme which emerged from the data was how relationships between educators and parents had changed, in part due to enforced changes in how people meet (in person to online) but also due to changes which have occurred more broadly across society. Some of these changes are perceived as positive (for instance, parents not coming into kindergarten buildings or rooms was mentioned by a surprisingly large number of respondents) while others are not so positive (distance between kindergarten staff and parents, lack of parental involvement). Negotiating these changes and cultivating professional relationships with parents will be vital to the ongoing viability as well as health of Steiner kindergartens.

Change and responsivity

The second theme is that of change and responsivity. The Covid-19 pandemic was an event beyond anyone's control. It has been possible to mitigate its impact in some ways, but it presented every country with situations which no one had experienced, and which demanded flexibility, adaptability and responsivity on a scale never needed before.

This was the case within Steiner education as well. What emerged strongly from the replies collected is the number of ways that Steiner educators have adapted to changing circumstances, often in ways they did not seek to or like, but which nonetheless have led to numerous practices being established which will be continued beyond the pandemic. Multiple

---

5 See Steiner's *Curative Course* (GA317), lecture 2.

respondents spoke to the strength of the pedagogy, how it could be adapted to meet the changed circumstances – indeed, there was no alternative. What it emphasised was the importance of the pedagogical moment, the moment of contact between child and teacher, to be forever renewed, no matter how challenging the circumstances.

While it is not possible to prepare for an unforeseen event, the pandemic highlights the importance of social and emotional learning to be part of all teacher education programmes. This is both to support children from a standpoint of knowledge and understanding, but also to meet the social and emotional needs of educators themselves. Trauma-informed pedagogy is becoming more established and more widely practised, including in Steiner circles. It would be worthwhile to make sure that aspects of this are included in all Steiner teacher education programmes, and that practising educators have opportunities to become familiar with it.

It is heartening and inspiring to read how staff in Steiner kindergartens have met the unprecedented challenges posed by the last three years, as they share their struggles and achievements, their highs and lows, successes and setbacks. There is a great deal which we do not know about the pandemic and what the long-term consequences for this generation of children will be. What I hope this report does, is open a small window into the lives of Steiner kindergartens around the world during September 2022. Through this window, we can hear educators, assistants, administrators and teacher educators speak of their experiences during this extraordinary time. I hope that hearing these voices from around the world will broaden the understanding of and feeling for the worldwide Steiner early childhood movement. So much of what we experienced of the pandemic has been personal within our local contexts. Hearing this chorus of voices can serve to broaden and enrich all of our understandings of the responses to and consequences of the Covid-19 pandemic on Steiner early childhood education.

Recommendations for future research

A simple definition of what research is, is to find out what was not known before and to share that knowledge and understanding with others. With this in mind, there are many topics raised by the current study which call for further treatment. A study which asks for responses from so many countries can serve to identify themes to be explored in depth in other, more specific, reports or articles.

Themes which merit further engagement include the whole topic of well-being which underpins much of this current study, the well-being of staff, of children, and of families. This could take the form of local or national anonymous reporting surveys which investigate the extent of and types of stressors all kindergarten staff experience, including steps towards their possible mitigation. Similarly, detailed examination of the incidence of anxiety and vulnerability in Steiner kindergarten children is called for, including pathways to ameliorate this which have proven successful in practice. The same is the case with reported speech and movement delay. These symptoms are widely reported across the education sector and numerous non-Steiner studies are underway. A research-informed response from the Steiner early childhood movement indicating how young children educated through the Covid pandemic can best be supported based on anthroposophical understandings of the young child would be of interest and benefit both within and beyond the Steiner early childhood community. This may be most fruitful if undertaken in conjunction with therapists and medical professionals.

It would be interesting to follow up with educators to see what their continued experience of modified practices is and if further amendments are made, or former practices and approaches begin to reassert themselves. Exploring new ways of working with parents and how staff strengthen links to parental communities could also be beneficial.

Many respondents wrote about divisions within their communities as variations of the vax/antivax debate. It would be important to see what can be learned from those kindergartens or national organisations who reported working successfully with this division to establish some form of best practice. Although these divisions may have lessened with the repeal of mandates, it is not unlikely that the fault lines could reopen in the future should another such unexpected event occur. There is also the issue of addressing reputational damage in some countries. Research into what proved helpful in this regard during the pandemic could also be helpful in the future.

An illuminating section of this report is to the question, 'what is the most import thing you have learned?' This merits much more detailed unpacking, as it illustrates processes undertaken and undergone by kindergarten staff during the pandemic. These avenues of transformation can be explored in many ways. What do German or US educators say their main learning is? Is it the same as their colleagues in Australia, Japan and Brazil? Is it the same as teacher educators? Have the insights gained proven helpful and been put into practice? If so, in which ways and to what effect? Will what has been learned help Waldorf early childhood to become more resilient and responsive in the future?

The question of leadership emerges in a few places during the report. It would be important to assess what helped and what did not really help during the pandemic period, should a similar situation ever occur again. What would have been beneficial which was not offered? What could have been done more? What could be done less? Communication was highlighted as key. Do structures need putting in place to facilitate this? How can well-being best be supported by leadership and organisations? This is undoubtedly of relevance to IASWECE as well as national bodies.

Lastly, it would be worthwhile studying in detail what has been learned from the pandemic experience so it can inform those who work in early childhood educator preparation and professional development programmes. This could take the form of interviews with current or past students and tutors, as well as surveys. Such knowledge would be valuable to gather and distribute so centres worldwide can learn from each other.

Strengths and limitations

Issues raised by participants are supported by prior research (outside of Steiner contexts) and public discourse, which suggests that the responses given reflect current issues in the early childhood sector on a wider scale (Jalongo, 2021).

Although participants' personal data were not collected, having responses from assistants, educators, administrators as well as those in teacher education guaranteed responses from those in different roles with different levels of experience. Future studies will be able to investigate the backgrounds of the participants further. The use of mixed methods in this study (quantitative as well as qualitative), helped ensure that data collected was rich and nuanced and represented a range of experiences from educators in very different locations.

A principal limitation of the study is that not all countries or continents are represented equally. This can be seen by the strongly varied rate of response in Table 4. However, this is offset to a degree by the overall number of responses from around the world. Many promising avenues of inquiry are indicated by this study which call out for further work.

Acknowledgements

I would like to acknowledge and thank the International Association for Steiner Waldorf Early Childhood Education (IASWECE), the Förderstiftung für Anthroposophische Medizin in Switzerland, the Waldorf Early Childhood Association of North America (WECAN) and Waekura New Zealand for funding to support this study, and to all those who helped with translations.

Thanks also to Dr Stefan Roesch for his advice regarding questionnaire design and Dr Aarthi Srinivasan for her assistance with the initial analysis of the text-based responses.

Lastly, I would like to give a personal word of thanks to Susan Howard from the Coordinating Group of IASWECE for her constant advice and support, and to Waldorf kindergarten staff around the world who took the time to complete the questionnaires.

Disclosure statement

No potential conflict of interest was reported by the author.

Correspondence

All correspondence regarding this report should be directed to Dr Neil Boland: neil.boland@aut.ac.nz

Appendices

Appendix A: Participant Information Sheet

Participant Information Sheet

Date Information Sheet Produced:

29 June 2022

Project Title

Covid-19 pandemic: Responses and consequences in Steiner Waldorf early childhood settings

An Invitation

My name is Neil Boland, and I am senior lecturer in the School of Education at Auckland University of Technology, New Zealand. I invite you to take part in a research project which looks at the effect of the Covid-19 pandemic in Steiner early childhood settings around the world.

What is the purpose of this research?

This research is being undertaken for IASWECE, the international Steiner early childhood body. It will gather information from Steiner early childhood educators about the responses to and consequences of the Covid-19 pandemic and their experiences during the subsequent learning period. It explores current levels of teacher, child and family wellbeing, if and how child development and teaching practices have been affected, as well as current challenges and needs.

From this research, a report will be produced which will be publicly available. A summary report will also be prepared and translated into the languages of IASWECE members. These will be able to be downloaded from the IASWECE website.

The findings of the research may also be used for further publications or presentations.

How was I identified and why am I being invited to participate in this research?

You have been identified as working in a Steiner early childhood setting. As a Steiner early childhood teacher/kindergartner, administrator, assistant teacher, or teacher educator, you are warmly invited to take part in the research.

How do I agree to participate in this research?

If you want to participate in this research, please click the links provided to the online questionnaires. The first screen of the questionnaire is a consent form. If you are happy to continue after reading the form, click 'I agree' at the foot of the page.

Your participation in this research is voluntary (it is your choice) and whether or not you choose to participate will neither advantage nor disadvantage you. You can leave the questionnaire at any time before the end. Once you have submitted your responses, your data can be neither identified nor withdrawn.

What will happen in this research?

The research takes the form of two online questionnaires. The first is short – you can complete it on your phone or on a laptop as you wish – and will take a few minutes. The second is separate and asks for more detailed responses. It is best completed on a laptop or similar and will take around half an hour. No personal information is collected, and your response is anonymous. Any data collected will be used for the purpose of this report to IASWECE and may also be used for other publications and outputs.

What are the discomforts and risks?

All responses in this project will be anonymous. No identifying data is asked for. I don't anticipate that there will be any risk associated with this research.

How will these discomforts and risks be alleviated?

If you find any questions uncomfortable, miss them out. You can stop and leave the questionnaire at any time. If you have concerns, see contacts below.

1 September 2022   page 1 of 2

COVID-19 pandemic: Responses and consequences in Steiner Waldorf early childhood settings

Text of Participant Information Sheet:

Date Information Sheet Produced:

29 June 2022

Project Title

Covid-19 pandemic: Responses and consequences in Steiner Waldorf early childhood settings

An Invitation

My name is Neil Boland, and I am senior lecturer in the School of Education at Auckland University of Technology, New Zealand. I invite you to take part in a research project which looks at the effect of the Covid-19 pandemic in Steiner early childhood settings around the world.

What is the purpose of this research?

This research is being undertaken for IASWECE, the international Steiner early childhood body. It will gather information from Steiner early childhood educators about the responses to and consequences of the Covid-19 pandemic and their experiences during the subsequent learning period. It explores current levels of teacher, child and family well-being, if and how child development and teaching practices have been affected, as well as current challenges and needs.

From this research, a report will be produced which will be publicly available. A summary report will also be prepared and translated into the languages of IASWECE members. These will be able to be downloaded from the IASWECE website.

The findings of the research may also be used for further publications or presentations.

How was I identified and why am I being invited to participate in this research?

You have been identified as working in a Steiner early childhood setting. As a Steiner early childhood teacher/kindergartner, administrator, assistant teacher, or teacher educator, you are warmly invited to take part in the research.

How do I agree to participate in this research?

If you want to participate in this research, please click the links provided to the online questionnaires. The first screen of the questionnaire is a consent form. If you are happy to continue after reading the form, click 'I agree' at the foot of the page.

Your participation in this research is voluntary (it is your choice) and whether or not you choose to participate will neither advantage nor disadvantage you. You can leave the questionnaire at any time before the end. Once you have submitted your responses, your data can be neither identified nor withdrawn.

What will happen in this research?

The research takes the form of two online questionnaires. The first is short – you can complete it on your phone or on a laptop as you wish – and will take a few minutes. The second is separate and asks for more detailed responses. It is best completed on a laptop or similar and will take around half an hour. No personal information is collected, and your response is anonymous. Any data collected will be used for the purpose of this report to IASWECE and may also be used for other publications and outputs.

What are the discomforts and risks?

All responses in this project will be anonymous. No identifying data is asked for. I don't anticipate that there will be any risk associated with this research.

How will these discomforts and risks be alleviated?

If you find any questions uncomfortable, miss them out. You can stop and leave the questionnaire at any time. If you have concerns, see contacts below.

What are the benefits?

This research aims to provide an overview of how the Steiner Waldorf early childhood movement as a whole has responded to and been affected by the Covid-19 pandemic. It hopes to identify innovative practices, attitudes to and consequences of the pandemic which can inform future action. The information is being gathered worldwide and will be collated for IASWECE to inform its future planning and actions. There is no personal benefit to you.

How will my privacy be protected?

The questionnaire is anonymous. No data will be collected which will enable anyone (including the researcher) to identify you or your place of employment. All results will be presented in aggregate rather than individual form.

What are the costs of participating in this research?

I anticipate that the short questionnaire will take five minutes of your time and the longer questionnaire around 30 minutes.

What opportunity do I have to consider this invitation?

After receiving this invitation, you will have until 30 September 2022 to complete the questionnaires.

Will I receive feedback on the results of this research?

From this research, a report will be written (in English) which will be available on the IASWECE website. A summary of the overall findings will also be available on the website in multiple languages.

What do I do if I have concerns about this research?

Any concerns regarding the nature of this project should be notified in the first instance to the Project Supervisor, *Dr Neil Boland, neil.boland@ aut.ac.nz, +649 921 9999 ext.7341.*

Concerns regarding the conduct of the research should be notified to the Executive Secretary of AUTEC, ethics@aut.ac.nz, +649 921 9999 ext. 6038.

Whom do I contact for further information about this research?

Please keep this Information Sheet for your future reference. You are also able to contact the research team as follows:

Researcher Contact Details:

Dr Neil Boland, neil.boland@aut.ac.nz, *+649 921 9999 ext.7341.*

Approved by the Auckland University of Technology Ethics Committee on 29 June 2022, AUTEC Reference number 22/166.

Appendix B: Invitation Letter

Dear colleagues,

IASWECE is undertaking some research into the response of Steiner early childhood settings to the Covid pandemic and its effects. It is being led by Dr Neil Boland of Auckland University of Technology in New Zealand. See the attached Information Sheet. Neil will write a report for IASWECE based on the information gathered which will give us an overview of how we as a worldwide body have responded to and been affected by the Covid-19 pandemic. It hopes to identify innovative practices and identify consequences of the pandemic which can inform future action. This is valuable information to have. He will also write a shorter summary report which will be available in multiple languages. These will be available on the IASWECE website. I will share the links with you when they are complete.

There are two questionnaires – one short which you can do on your phones in five minutes, and a longer one which will be easiest on a laptop and will take around 30 minutes to complete.

Please encourage everyone in your centres to complete the first questionnaire – it will just take a few minutes. You can do it on your phones. The second questionnaire takes longer and asks for more thoughtful, detailed responses. The information is being gathered in IASWECE member countries all over the world.

Quick questionnaire 1

https://aut.au1.qualtrics.com/jfe/form/SV_d4OrEqP0RX4y9Js

Longer questionnaire 2

https://aut.au1.qualtrics.com/jfe/form/SV_6gs9LYFZGH3DC8m

I am attaching an information sheet which explains it in detail. By submitting the questionnaire, you consent to taking part in this aspect of the research.

Centre leaders – please send this email to all your teachers, assistant teachers and to mentor settings if you have them, for them to share with their teachers. You may like to make time in your next meeting to talk about this and for teachers to complete the shorter questionnaire during the meeting (on their phones). The more responses we get, the richer the information we can gather. The questionnaires will be open for the month of September.

This is the first global research project which IASWECE has undertaken.

Please help by encouraging as many people as possible to respond, especially to the first questionnaire!

With warm greetings,

Appendix C: Questionnaire 1

Covid-19 pandemic: Responses and consequences in Steiner Waldorf early childhood settings

Questionnaire 1

My name is Neil Boland and I am senior lecturer in the School of Education at Auckland University of Technology, New Zealand. I invite you to take part in a small research project which looks at effects of the Covid-19 pandemic in Steiner early childhood settings around the world.

What is the purpose of this research?

This research is being undertaken for IASWECE, the international Steiner early childhood body. It seeks to gather information from Steiner early childhood educators about the responses to and consequences of the Covid-19 pandemic and their experiences of the subsequent learning period. From this research, a report will be produced which will be publicly available.

What will happen in this research?

This anonymous questionnaire will take around 5 minutes. It can be completed on a phone or laptop as you wish. Any data collected will be used for the purpose of this report to IASWECE and may also be used for other publications and outputs. By submitting the questionnaire, you agree to take part in this aspect of the research project.

How do I agree to participate in this research?

If you want to participate in this research, read these statements and, if you agree with them, please check the box below.

- I have read and understood the information provided about this research project in the Information Sheet dated 29 June 2022.
- I understand that taking part in this questionnaire is voluntary (my choice) and that whether or not I participate will not disadvantage me in any way.
- I understand that I can leave the questionnaire at any time before the end and that once I have submitted the responses, my data can be neither identified nor withdrawn.

Approved by the Auckland University of Technology Ethics Committee on 29 June 2022. AUTEC Reference number 22/166.

☐ *I agree with the statements above and wish to take part in this research project*

What is your main professional role?

- Early childhood teacher/ educator/ kindergartner
- Teacher assistant
- Administrator
- Administrator and teacher
- Work in teacher education

WELL-BEING

How do you rate the following, compared to before the pandemic:

Your well-being as a teacher

- Much better
- Moderately better
- Slightly better
- About the same
- Slightly worse
- Moderately worse
- Much worse

The well-being of their families

- Much better
- Moderately better
- Slightly better
- About the same
- Slightly worse
- Moderately worse
- Much worse

The well-being of children in your care

- Much better
- Moderately better
- Slightly better
- About the same
- Slightly worse
- Moderately worse
- Much worse

The well-being of your colleagues

- Much better
- Moderately better
- Slightly better
- About the same
- Slightly worse
- Moderately worse
- Much worse

The well-being of the society you live in

- Much better
- Moderately better
- Slightly better
- About the same
- Slightly worse
- Moderately worse
- Much worse

The well-being of the parent community

- Much better
- Moderately better
- Slightly better
- About the same
- Slightly worse
- Moderately worse
- Much worse

Your own well-being

- Much better
- Moderately better
- Slightly better
- About the same
- Slightly worse
- Moderately worse
- Much worse

CHILD DEVELOPMENT

Compared to before the pandemic, how would you rate the incidence among children of the following:

Speech delay

- Much less common
- A little less common
- More or less the same
- A little more common
- Much more common

Movement delay

- Much less common
- A little less common
- More or less the same
- A little more common
- Much more common

General vulnerability

- Much less common
- A little less common
- More or less the same
- A little more common
- Much more common

Anxiety attending EC centre

- Much less common
- A little less common
- More or less the same
- A little more common
- Much more common

Separation anxiety

- Much less common
- A little less common
- More or less the same
- A little more common
- Much more common

Willingness to share with others

- Much less common
- A little less common
- More or less the same
- A little more common
- Much more common

Fear of groups

- Much less common
- A little less common
- More or less the same
- A little more common
- Much more common

General anxiety

- Much less common
- A little less common
- More or less the same
- A little more common
- Much more common

ENROLMENT AND STAFFING

Compared to before the pandemic:

Number of children on the roll

- Much higher
- A little higher
- More or less the same
- A little lower
- Much lower

Staff turnover (compared to other periods)

- Much higher
- A little higher
- More or less the same
- A little lower
- Much lower

Number of children attending regularly

- Much higher
- A little higher
- More or less the same
- A little lower
- Much lower

Inquiries and enrolments

- Much higher
- A little higher
- More or less the same
- A little lower
- Much lower

Has your organisation been negatively affected by vaccine mandates?

- Not applicable
- Not affected negatively
- Slightly negative
- Moderately negative
- Strongly negative

Powered by Qualtrics

Appendix D: Questionnaire 2

Covid-19 pandemic: Responses and consequences in Steiner Waldorf early childhood settings

Questionnaire 2

My name is Neil Boland and I am senior lecturer in the School of Education at Auckland University of Technology, New Zealand. I invite you to take part in a small research project which looks at effects of the Covid-19 pandemic in Steiner early childhood settings around the world.

What is the purpose of this research?

This anonymous questionnaire will take around 30 minutes. It is best completed on a laptop. Any data collected will be used for the purpose of this report to IASWECE and may also be used for other publications and outputs.

What will happen in this research?

This anonymous questionnaire will take around 30 minutes. It can be completed on a phone or laptop as you wish. Any data collected will be used for the purpose of this report to IASWECE and may also be used for other publications and outputs. By submitting the questionnaire, you agree to take part in this aspect of the research project.

How do I agree to participate in this research?

If you want to participate in this research, read these statements and, if you agree with them, please check the box below.

- I have read and understood the information provided about this research project in the Information Sheet dated 29 June 2022.
- I understand that taking part in this questionnaire is voluntary (my choice) and that whether or not I participate will not disadvantage me in any way.
- I understand that I can leave the questionnaire at any time before the end and that once I have submitted the responses, my data can be neither identified nor withdrawn.

Approved by the Auckland University of Technology Ethics Committee on 29 June 2022. AUTEC Reference number 22/166.

☐ *I agree with the statements above and wish to take part in this research project*

What is your main professional role?

- Early childhood teacher/ educator/ kindergartner
- Teacher assistant
- Administrator
- Administrator and teacher
- Work in teacher education

This survey contains only four questions. Please take your time to answer them fully, and reflectively. The more detail you are able to provide, the more helpful your answers will be. Thank you.

1. Which of the changes you have made to your practice during the pandemic will you keep, and why?
2. How have you viewed Waldorf early childhood education during these pandemic experiences? (Strengths / things to change)
3. What is the most important thing you have learned from the pandemic experience?
4. What is the single greatest challenge you face?

Powered by Qualtrics

References

AFP. (2021, December 23). *A spiritual movement and Germany's low vaccination rate*. France24. https://www.france24.com/en/live-news/20211123-a-spiritual-movement-and-germany-s-low-vaccination-rate

Atiles, J. T., Almodóvar, M., Vargas, A. C., Dias, M. J. A., & León, I. M. Z. (2022). International responses to COVID-19: Challenges faced by early childhood professionals. *European Early Childhood Education Research Journal,, 29*(1), 66-78. https://doi.org/https://doi.org/10.1080/1350293X.2021.1872674

Attfield, K. (2022). The young child's journey of 'the will': A synthesis of child-centered and inclusive principles in international Waldorf early childhood education. *Journal of Early Childhood Research, 20*(2), 159–171. https://doi.org/https://doi.org/https://doi.org/10.1038/s41598-022-05840-5

Bergmann, C., Dimitrova, N., Alaslani, K., Almohammadi, A., Alroqi, H., Aussems, S., Barokova, M., Davies, C., Gonzalez-Gomez, N., Gibson, S. P., Havron, N., Horowitz-Kraus, T., Kanero, J., Kartushina, N., Keller, C., Mayor, J., Mundry, R., Shinskey, J., & Mani , N. (2022). Young children's screen time during the first COVID-19 lockdown in 12 countries. *Scientific Reports, 22*(2015). https://doi.org/https://doi.org/10.1038/s41598-022-05840-5

Bernardi, L., & Gotlib, I. H. (2022). COVID-19 stressors, mental/emotional distress and political support. *West European Politics, 46*(2), 425-436. https://doi.org/https://doi.org/10.1080/01402382.2022.2055372

Boland, N. (2020a). *Responses to Covid-19 restrictions in Steiner early childhood settings in Australia.* Auckland University of Technology. https://www.goetheanum-paedagogik.ch/fileadmin/paedagogik/Artikel/Response_of_Steiner_ECE_to_Covid_restrictions_in_Australia_FINAL.pdf

Boland, N. (2020b). *Responses to Covid-19 restrictions in Steiner early childhood settings: A comparison of Australian and New Zealand experiences.* Auckland University of Technology. https://www.goetheanum-paedagogik.ch/fileadmin/paedagogik/Artikel/Covid-19_restrictions_in_Steiner_centres_in_Australia_and_New_Zealand_FINAL.pdf

Boland, N., & Mortlock, A. (2020). *Responses to Covid-19 in Steiner early childhood settings in New Zealand.* Auckland University of Technology. https://www.goetheanum-paedagogik.ch/fileadmin/paedagogik/Artikel/Response_of_Steiner_ECE_to_Covid_restrictions_in_NZ_FINAL.pdf

Braun, V., Clarke, V., Hayfield, N., & Terry, G. (2018). Thematic analysis. In P. Liamputtong (Ed.), *Handbook of Research Methods in Health Social Sciences,* (pp. 1-18). Springer Nature. https://doi.org/10.1007/978-981-10-2779-6_103-1

Byström, E., Lindstrand, A., Likhite, N., Butler, R., & Emmelin, M. (2014). Parental attitudes and decision-making regarding MMR vaccination in an anthroposophic community in Sweden – A qualitative study. *Vaccine, 32*(50), 6752-6757. https://doi.org/10.1016/j.vaccine.2014.10.011

Croasmun, J. T., & Ostrom, L. (2011). Using Likert-type scales in the social sciences. *Journal of Adult Education, 40*(1), 19-22.

Cumming, T. (2017). Early childhood educators' well-being: An updated review of the literature. *Early Childhood Education Journal, 45*(5), 583–593. https://doi.org/10.1007/s10643-016-0818-6

de Souza, D. L. (2012). Learning and human development in Waldorf pedagogy and curriculum. *Encounter, 25*(4), 50-62.

Doetter, L. F., Preuß, B., & Frisina, P. G. (2022). The intersections of pandemic, public policy and social inequality in the United States. *Forum for Social Economics, 5*(1), 220-223. https://doi.org/https://doi.org/10.1080/07360932.2021.1967182

Eadie, P., Levickis, P., Murray, L., Page, J., Elek, C., & Church, A. (2021). Early childhood educators' wellbeing during the COVID-19 pandemic. *Early Childhood Education Journal 49*, 903–913. https:// doi.org/https://doi.org/10.1007/s10643-021-01203-3

Ejsing, M., & Denman, D. (2022). Democratic politics in virulent times: Three vital lessons from the COVID-19 pandemic. *Distinktion: Journal of Social Theory*. https://doi.org/https://doi.org/10.1080/1600910X.2022.2054448

Escritt, T. (2021, February 10). *Wealthy German high-tech hub doubles as anti-vaxxer base*. Reuters. https://www.reuters.com/article/us-health-coronavirus-germany-anti-vacci-idUSKBN2A91KQ

Esposito, S., & Principi, N. (2020). To mask or not to mask children to overcome COVID-19. *European Journal of Pediatrics, 179*, 1267–1270. https://doi.org/https://doi.org/10.1007/s00431-020-03674-9

Farina, M., & Lavazza, A. (2021). The meaning of Freedom after Covid-19. *History and Philosophy of the Life Sciences, 43*(3). https:// doi.org/https://doi.org/10.1007/s40656-020-00354-7

Farrer, M. (2020, October 8). *New Zealand's Covid-19 response the best in the world, say global business leaders*. https://www.theguardian.com/ world/2020/oct/08/new-zealands-covid-19-response-the-best-in-the-world-say-global-business-leaders

Fegert, J. M., Vitiello, B., Plener, P. L., & Clemens, V. (2020). Challenges and burden of the Coronavirus 2019 (COVID-19) pandemic for child and adolescent mental health: A narrative review to highlight clinical and research needs in the acute phase and the long return to normality. *Child and Adolescent Psychiatry and Mental Health, 14*(20). https://doi.org/https://doi.org/10.1186/s13034-020-00329-3

Flack, C. B., Walker, L., Bickerstaff, A., & Margetts, C. (2020). *Socioeconomic disparities in Australian schooling during the Covid-19 pandemic*. Pivot Professional Learning.

Flaherty, C. (2022, June 13). *The peer-review crisis*. Inside Higher Ed. https://www.insidehighered.com/news/2022/06/13/peer-review-crisis-creates-problems-journals-and-scholars

Foord, C. (2022). *A program evaluation of the impact of COVID-19 on teacher mobility, attrition, and retentionmobility, attrition, and retention* National Louis University]. Chicago, IL. https://digitalcommons.nl.edu/cgi/viewcontent. cgi?article=1685&context=diss

Foucault, M., Davidson, A. I., & Burchell, G. (2008). *The birth of biopolitics: Lectures at the Collège de France, 1978–1979.* Springer.

Freunde der Erziehungskunst Rudolf Steiners. (2022). *Waldorf world list.* Retrieved August 27 from https://www.freunde-waldorf.de/fileadmin/user_upload/images/Waldorf_World_List/Waldorf_World_List.pdf

Gauthier, G. R., Smith, J. A., García, C., Garcia, M. A., & Thomas, P. A. (2020). Exacerbating inequalities: Social networks, racial/ethnic disparities, and the Covid-19 pandemic in the United States. *Journals of Gerontology, Series B,* gbaa117. https://doi.org/10.1093/geronb/gbaa117

Gillespie, A., & Breen, C. (2021, November 5). *Protesting in a pandemic: New Zealand's balancing act between a long tradition of protests and Covid rules.* The Conversation. https://www.rnz.co.nz/news/national/455026/protesting-in-a-pandemic-new-zealand-s-balancing-act-between-a-long-tradition-of-protests-and-covid-rules

Greyling, T., Rossouw, S., & Adhikari, T. (2021). A tale of three countries: What is the relationship between Covid-19, lockdown and happiness? *South African Journal of Economics, 81*(1), 25-41. https://doi.org/doi: 10.1111/saje.12284

Guest, G., MacQueen, K. M., & Namey, E. E. (2012). Introduction to applied thematic analysis. In G. Guest, K. M. MacQueen, & E. E. Namey (Eds.), *Applied thematic analysis.* Sage. https://doi.org/10.4135/9781483384436

Haelermans, C., Korthals, R., Jacobs, M., Leeuw, S. d., Vermeulen, S., Vugt, L. v., Aarts, B., Prokic-Breuer, T., Velden, R. v. d., Wetten, S. v., & Wolf, I. d. (2022). Sharp increase in inequality in education in times of the COVID-19-pandemic. *PLoS ONE, 17*(2), e0261114. https://doi.org/10.1371/journal.pone.0261114

Henry, A. J. L., Hatfield, B. E., & Chandler, K. D. (2021). Toddler teacher job strain, resources, and classroom quality. *International Journal of Early Years Education,* 1-15. https://doi.org/10.1080/09669760.2021.1892596

Herbert, B., MacKenzie, B., & Saunders, M. (2021). *Mullumbimby Steiner school loses 40 staff over COVID-19 vaccination deadline.* ABC News. https://www.abc.net.au/news/2021-11-07/mullumbimby-steiner-shearwater-teachers-unvaccinated/100600130

Hinsliff, G. (2022, January 29). *'My son cowers when a shopkeeper says hello' – are the toddlers of Covid all right?* https://www.theguardian.com/world/2022/jan/29/my-son-cowers-when-a-shopkeeper-says-hello-are-the-toddlers-of-covid-all-right

Huppertz, H. I., Berner, R., Schepke, r. R., Kopp, M., Oberle, A., Fischbach, T., Rodeck, B., Knuf, M., Keller, M., Simon, A., & Hübner, J. (2021). Use of masks by children to prevent infection with SARS-CoV-2. *Monatsschrift Kinderheilkunde: Organ der Deutschen Gesellschaft fur Kinderheilkunde, 169*(1), 52–56. https://doi.org/ https://doi.org/10.1007/s00112-020-01090-9

International Federation of Anthroposophic Medical Associations (IVAA) and the Medical Section of the Goetheanum. (2021, January 12). *Anthroposophic medicine statement on vaccination against SARS-CoV-2* https://www.salutogenesi.org/approfondimenti/salute/anthroposophic-medicine-statement-on-vaccination-against-sars-cov-2

Jalongo, M. R. (2021). The effects of COVID19 on early childhood education and care: Research and resources for children, families, teachers, and teacher educators. *Early Childhood Education Journal, 49*, 763–774. https://doi.org/https://doi.org/10.1007/s10643-021-01208-y

James, N., Neilson, M., & Weekes, J. (2022, March 3). *Covid 19 Wellington protest: Riots, fire and violence as police end occupation.* New Zealand Herald. https://www.nzherald.co.nz/nz/politics/covid-19-wellington-protest-riots-fire-and-violence-as-police-end-occupation/SKA5WAE3HBT3GZOY2SNZPOBWLY/

Jones, J. (2020). *Getting it right: Using implementation research to improve outcomes in early care and education.* https://www.fcd-us.org/assets/2020/06/GettingitRight_UsingImplementationResearchtoImproveOutcomesinECE_2020.pdf

Kasstan, B. (2021). Vaccines and vitriol: an anthropological commentary on vaccine hesitancy, decision-making and interventionism among religious minorities. *Anthropology & Medicine, 28*(4), 411-419. https://doi.org/https://www.tandfonline.com/action/showCitFormats?doi=10.1080/13648470.2020.1825618

Kwon, K.-A., Malek, A., Horm, D., & Castle, S. (2020). Turnover and retention of infant-toddler teachers: Reasons, consequences, and implications for practice and policy. *Children and Youth Services Review, 115.* https://doi.org/10.1016/j.childyouth.2020.105061

Lafave, L., Webster, A. D., & McConnell, C. (2022). Impact of COVID-19 on early childhood educator's perspectives and practices in nutrition and physical activity: A qualitative study. *Early Childhood Education Journal 49*, 935–945. https://doi.org/https://doi.org/10.1007/s10643-021-01195-0

Mayring, P. (2020). Qualitative content analysis: Demarcation, varieties, developments. *Forum: Qualitative Social Research, 20*(3). https://doi.org/http://dx.doi.org/10.17169/fqs-20.3.3343

McClure, T. (2022, February 25). 'So many rabbit holes': Even in trusting New Zealand, protests show fringe beliefs can flourish. The Guardian. https://www.theguardian.com/world/2022/feb/26/so-many-rabbit-holes-even-in-trusting-new-zealand-protests-show-fringe-beliefs-can-flourish

McFarland, L., Cumming, T., Wong, S., & Bull, R. (2022). 'My cup was empty': The impact of COVID-19 on early childhood educator well-being. In J. Pattnaik & M. R. Jalongo (Eds.), *The impact of COVID-19 on early childhood education and care* (pp. 171-192). Springer. https://doi.org/https://doi.org/10.1007/978-3-030-96977-6_9#DOI

Medical Section at the Goetheanum. (2019, April 14). *Anthroposophic medicine statement on vaccination.* Medical Section of the Goetheanum and the International Federation of Anthroposophic Medical Associations,. Retrieved October 11 from https://www.ivaa.info/latest-news/article/article/anthroposophic-medicine-statement-on-vaccination/

Mensch, C. (2021, December 23). *Rudolf Steiner Schule Basel: Shitstorm nach missglückter Masken-Kommunikation.* Basellandschaftliche Zeitung.

Mitchell, L., Hodgen, E., Meagher-Lundberg, P., & Wells, C. (2020). *Impact of Covid-19 on the early childhood education sector in Aotearoa New Zealand: Challenges and opportunities. Initial findings from a survey of managers.* Wilf Malcolm Institute of Educational Research.

Molyneux, V. (2021, August 27). *Majority of New Zealand supports COVID-19 lockdown - research.* https://www.newshub.co.nz/home/new-zealand/2021/08/majority-of-new-zealand-supports-covid-19-lockdown-research.html

New Zealand Herald. (2022, March 3). *Covid 19 Wellington protest: World reacts to Wellington protesters setting 'Parliament lawn ablaze'*. New Zealand Herald. https://www.nzherald.co.nz/nz/covid-19-wellington-protest-world-reacts-to-wellington-protesters-setting-parliament-lawn-ablaze/TGS7XT4GBPEOFJCPHXB3YAAMNQ/

Nicol, J., & Taplin, T. J. (2017). *Understanding the Steiner Waldorf approach: Early years education in practice* (2nd ed.). Routledge.

Noble, K., Hurley, P., & Macklin, S. (2020). *COVID-19, employment stress and student vulnerability in Australia*. www.mitchellinstitute.org.au

NSW Government. (2020, August 17). *Updated COVID-Safe guidelines for NSW schools*. NSW Government. Retrieved October 10 from https://education.nsw.gov.au/news/latest-news/updated-covid-safe-guidelines-for-nsw-schools

O'Connor, D., & Angus, J. (2014). Give Them Time: An analysis of school readiness in Ireland's early education system: A Steiner Waldorf Perspective. *Education 3-13: International Journal of Primary, Elementary and Early Years Education, 42*(5), 488-497. https://doi.org/10.1080/03004279.2012.723726

O'Neill, G. P. (1986). Teacher education or teacher training: Which is it? *McGill Journal of Education, 22*(3), 257-265.

Osgood, J. (2021). In pursuit of worldly justice in Early Childhood Education: Bringing critique and creation into productive partnership for the public good. In A. Ross (Ed.), *Educational Research for Social Justice* (Vol. 1, pp. 171–188). Springer. https://doi.org/https://doi.org/10.1007/978-3-030-62572-6_8

Oxford University Blavatnik School of Government. (2022). *Coronavirus government response tracker*. Retrieved November 14 from https://www.bsg.ox.ac.uk/research/research-projects/coronavirus-government-response-tracker#data

Patten, M. L. (2017). *Questionnaire research: A practical guide* (4th ed.). Routledge.

Press, F., Woodrow, C., Logan, H., & Mitchell, L. (2018). Can we belong in a neo-liberal world? Neo-liberalism in early childhood education and care policy in Australia and New Zealand. *Contemporary Issues in Early Childhood, 19*(4), 328-339. https://doi.org/10.1177/1463949118781909

Radanović, A., Micić, I., Pavlović, S., & Krstić, K. (2021). Don't think that kids aren't noticing: Indirect pathways to children's fear of COVID-19. *Frontiers in Psychology, 12*, 632952.

Randoll, D., & Peters, J. (2015). Empirical research on Waldorf education. *Educar em Revista, 56*, 33-47. https://doi.org/10.1590/01044060.41416

Rawson, M. (2021). *Steiner Waldorf pedagogy in schools: A critical introduction.* Routledge.

Redaelli, S. (2020, August 4). *Covid-19 and the perception of freedom.* Open Democracy. https://www.opendemocracy.net/en/can-europe-make-it/covid-19-and-perception-freedom/

Roberts-Holmes, G., & Moss, P. (2021). *Neoliberalism and early childhood education: Markets, imaginaries and governance.* Routledge.

Sancho, N. B., Mondragon, N. I., Santamaria, M. D., & Munitis, A. E. (2021). The Well-being of children in lock-down: Physical, emotional, social and academic impact. *Children and Youth Services Review, 127*. https://doi.org/10.1016/j.childyouth.2021.106085

Schifferes, S. (2020, April 10). *The coronavirus pandemic is already increasing inequality.* The Conversation. https://theconversation.com/the-coronavirus-pandemic-is-already-increasing-inequality-135992

Schwarz, S., Jenetzky, E., Kraffta, H., Maurera, T., & Martin, D. (2021). Corona children studies "Co-Ki": First Results of a Germany-wide registry on mouth and nose covering (mask) in children. *Monatsschrift Kinderheilkunde, 169*(4), 353-364. https://doi.org/https://doi.org/10.21203/rs.3.rs-124394/v4

Selg, P. (2021, February). *Anthroposophy and right-wing extremism? The conduct of the Waldorf schools in the "Third Reich".* Erziehungskunst. https://www.erziehungskunst.de/en/news/spotlight/anthroposophy-and-right-wing-extremism-the-conduct-of-the-waldorf-schools-in-the-third-reich/

Shergold, P., Broadbent, J., Marshall, I., & Varghese, P. (2022). *An independent review into Australia's response to COVID-19.* E. INSTITUTE.

Siraj, I., Arancibia, V., & Barón, J. (2022). The role of management, leadership, and monitoring in producing quality learning outcomes in early childhood education. In M. Bendini & A. Devercelli (Eds.), *Quality early learning: Nurturing children's potential* (pp. 199-238). World Bank Publications. https://doi.org/https://doi.org/10.1596/978-1-4648-1795-3_ch5

Sobo, E. J. (2015). Social cultivation of vaccine refusal and delay among Waldorf (Steiner) school parents. *Medical Anthropology Quarterly, 29*(3), 381-399. https://doi.org/10.1111/maq.12214

Sobo, E. J. (2016). Theorizing (vaccine) refusal: Through the looking glass. *Cultural Anthropology, 31*(3), 342–350. https://doi.org/10.14506/ca31.3.04

Souto-Manninga, M., & Melvina, S. A. (2022). Early childhood teachers of color in New York City: heightened stress, lower quality of life, declining health, and compromised sleep amidst COVID-19. *Early Childhood Research Quarterly, 60,* 38-48. https://doi.org/https://doi.org/10.1016/j.ecresq.2021.11.005

Sparks, S. D. (2022, November 15). *Pandemic anxiety was higher for teachers than for health-care workers.* EducationWeek. https://www.edweek.org/teaching-learning/pandemic-anxiety-was-higher-for-teachers-than-for-health-care-workers/2022/11

Stajduhar, A., Ganel, T., Avidan, G., Rosenbaum, R. S., & Freud, E. (2022). Face masks disrupt holistic processing and face perception in school-age children. *Cognitive Research: Principles and Implications 7*(9). https://doi.org/https://doi.org/10.1186/s41235-022-00360-2

Steiner, R. (1924/1998). *Education for special needs: The curative education course* [GA317]. Rudolf Steiner Press.

Su, J., Ng, D. T. K., Yang, W., & Li, H. (2022). Global trends in the research on early childhood education during the COVID-19 pandemic: A bibliometric analysis *education sciences, 12*(331). https://doi.org/https://doi.org/10.3390/educsci12050331

Tatsiopoulou, P., Holeva, V., Nikopoulou, V.-A., Parlapani, E., & Diakogiannis, I. (2022). Children's anxiety and parenting self-efficacy during the COVID-19-related home confinement. *Child: Care, Health and Development, 48*(6), 1103-1111. https://doi.org/https://doi.org/10.1111/cch.13041

Timmins, B., & Thomas, D. (2022, January 20). *Inflation: Seven reasons the cost of living is going up around the world*. BBC. https://www.bbc.com/news/business-59982702

Timmons, K., Cooper, A., Bozek, E., & Braund, H. (2021). The impacts of COVID19 on early childhood education: Capturing the unique challenges associated with remote teaching and learning in K2. *Early Childhood Education Journal, 49*, 887–901. https://doi.org/https://doi.org/10.1007/s10643-021-01207-z

Totenhagen, C. J., Hawkins, S. A., Casper, D. M., Bosch, L. A., Hawkey, K. R., & Borden, L. M. (2016). Retaining early childhood education workers: A review of the empirical literature. *Journal of Research In Childhood Education, 30*(4), 585–599. https://doi.org/http://dx.doi.org/10.1080/02568543.2016.1214652

Victoria University of Wellington. (2020, 24 June). *Lockdown survey finds NZ families 'incredibly robust', despite economic jolt*. Roy McKenzie Centre for the Study of Families and Children. Retrieved September 24 from https://www.wgtn.ac.nz/rmc/news/lockdown-survey-finds-nz-families-incredibly-robust,-despite-economic-jolt

Viola, T. W., & Nunes, M. L. (2022). Social and environmental effects of the COVID-19 pandemic on children. *Jornal de Pediatria, 98*(1), 4-12. https://doi.org/https://doi.org/10.1016/j.jped.2021.08.003

Will, M. (2021, September 24). *Some teachers won't get vaccinated, even with a mandate. What should schools do about it?* Education Week. https://www.edweek.org/leadership/some-teachers-wont-get-vaccinated-even-with-a-mandate-what-should-schools-do-about-it/2021/09

www.ingramcontent.com/pod-product-compliance
Lightning Source LLC
Chambersburg PA
CBHW060241030426
42335CB00014B/1561